BINGE EATING

Make Peace With Food

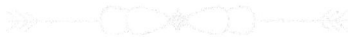

SIMON GRANT & SOPHIA DURNER

Table of Contents

Introduction

I know first-hand what having your own body and mind as your worst enemy feels like. I've had an unhealthy relationship with food ever since I was a child, and I can't say I'm proud of that. But things are better now. I am better, and with a little bit of help, I know that you can be better too.

If you're reading this book, that means that either you or someone that you care about are suffering from Binge-Eating Disorder. I will share my story with you, I'll show you the way out of this wreckage, and I'll walk by you each step of the way.

I know that some of you may have lost hope. I swear that there were times when I felt completely hopeless. I felt like I was watching myself eating from the outside, like a scene from a horror movie, as footage of an unstoppable disaster was happening before my eyes. Sometimes the guilt I felt afterward was so bad that I even wanted to die. My life was a disaster, and it all seemed so unfair. I was lost in a dark cave, and I couldn't see the way out.

Nonetheless, I can proudly say that I can see the light now. There was a way out of there, and I was able to regain control over myself slowly. I no longer feel as if my own body and mind are working against me, and if there was hope for me, trust me, there is hope for you too.

I've placed only the recommendations and strategies that actually helped me in this book. I can't be 100% sure that this will work with everyone because we are not all the same, but I would have loved to have someone on my side to tell me everything that I'm going to share with you when I needed it.

I also did a lot of study about this disease. Things are a lot different now as it has been recognized by the DSM 5, and there's a lot more information about it. I have studied this subject thoroughly, and I will give you the best tools that I found there - tools I wished I had at the beginning of it all.

With no further delay, let's get to the bottom of this, and by the end of this book, I'll meet you on the other side.

And I assure you, the view is far nicer from here.

Chapter One

Get to Know Me

First of all, let's start by letting you know who I am. My name is Sophia Durner. I am 32 years old and have a husband and two beautiful daughters, and I've been living in California for my whole life. I am 5'6" tall, and I weigh 165 pounds, so you know what this means. I have a potbelly, a double chin, fat legs, and arms with that disgusting fat that lingers underneath, and I have love handle after love handle stacked at both sides of my body. I know how I look. I'm well aware of it, and I've always been aware of it, but this is something that we'll look into in this book, so let's not get ahead of ourselves just yet.

I'm a teacher. I've always wanted to work around children, and now I can say this is my true calling. I love teaching, I love kids, I love my daughters, and I love the way I'm like a second mother to my students. It's true that I don't make a lot of money, but my husband works in the IT industry, so we're able to live a comfortable life.

I come from a large family. I grew up around the smell of homemade food, the mess caused by brawls between siblings, and the music my father used to play for us every now and then. I can't say I had an awful childhood; I know that I'm luckier than most people in the world, and I can't complain about financial shortages, but that doesn't mean everything was perfect. I'm the third of four sisters. Since I'm the only one who's overweight, I'm ashamed to say that I've always felt like the ugly duckling of the family. This is a story so common that you've probably heard it lots of times, but for me, it is the truth, and I know this may also be the truth for some of you.

My mother is a really great cook, and my childhood memories are tainted by the smell of food. Food has always meant a great deal to me. It was not only my nourishment, but it also provided peace, happiness, and that warm feeling that I've always related to my home. Being honest, maybe this had something to do with the development of Binge-Eating Disorder, but I'm no expert, and even if it had, maybe your stories are completely different, and your disease developed in a whole different way. The food my mother gave me made me feel great, and at times, it seemed like it was the only thing I had going in my life, so I believe it was a form of affection for me. What I do know for sure is what my therapist told me about myself definitely had something to do with it, and this was my low self-esteem due to my body weight.

As I've previously stated, I'm overweight. I've been fat ever since I was a girl. If you add this to the fact that I'm more of an introvert, you'll be able to guess how popular I was in school. I was a victim of bullying all the way from middle school to high school. Not only did I have my sisters to remind me of how different I was from them, but I was also made fun of because of my weight every single day in school. I still struggle with self-esteem issues, but things are better now. I have lost some of that weight, and I'm still going lower on the scale. Besides, I've come to change my mindset. Being overweight is no longer such a huge deal for me. We shouldn't value ourselves by the numbers displayed by our scale. Human beings are so much more than that, and this is something that you'll learn how to do later on in the book.

I'm only telling you this because I want you to understand me and, more importantly, if you feel like any bit of my story resembles yours, I want you to feel like you're not alone. This was a very important part of my therapy, and I feel like it really helped me, finally understanding that I am not alone.

I started Binge-Eating when I was around fourteen years old. My parents used to think that the snacks that disappeared from the kitchen cabinets were because of the four of us. The truth was that I used to grab these snacks, take them to my room, and wolf them down while reading books or watching the TV. At first, I did this whenever I had a rough day in school. Then I started doing it when I was bored, or something made me feel bad, or I did some overthinking until I was in a bad mood, among many different reasons. Soon I realized that I was unable to control it. My bodyweight went uphill, my self-esteem went lower as I saw my hips grow wider, and my belly grows larger, and the worse I felt about myself, the less I could control each binge-eating episode.

So, there you have it. This is where my story begins. I am a school teacher, a wife, and mother. I'm a sister and, most importantly, I'm a

Binge-Eating survivor. Right now, I'm the author of this book, and I will be your guide as we get you out of the same maze that I was in.

And we're going to go through it together.

Chapter Two

My Darkest Time

I started Binge-Eating when I was around fourteen years old. I was already overweight, I was an introvert, and my classmates were giving me a hard time over that. Every day I would hear people laughing behind my back, people stared at me with burlesque expressions on their faces, and they mostly avoided me, as if I was some sort of leper. I was able to survive mostly thanks to my best friend. Her name was Susan, and she was an angel sent by the heavens to take care of me.

Susan and I used to sit together during lunch break. We talked about the books we were reading, and we kept each other company during recess. She was my friend since fifth grade. She was the only one who showed me some kindness in the school, and I'll be forever grateful for it. Sadly, she wasn't very popular, either. Nevertheless, I guess you could say that at least we had each other. That was the truth until ninth grade when her father was transferred to Indiana, and she had to leave my school. I was devastated, and I already had a rough time with myself. Things were already bad for me, and suddenly I had to face school on my own.

Obviously, my Binge-Eating episodes got worse. It is hard to be a teenager. It's harder to be a teenager who's a victim of bullying, so you'll have to imagine what it's like to go through this by yourself. Some of you, sadly, don't need to imagine it. Some of us suffering from Binge-Eating Disorder had to go through very similar hardships. I guess you could say it's a part of life, but that doesn't mean it's easy, or fair. The fact is that I was alone, and that's when my binge urges started to strike harder, and my defenses were lower.

My first binge-eating episodes weren't that big. Maybe I made one or two popcorn bags in the microwave, mixed them in a bowl with cheese, crackers, sometimes cereal, and ate it while reading in my room. Sometimes I made myself three or four peanut butter and jelly sandwiches. Some other times I bought about one or two packages of Oreo cookies and ate them all at once. This was something that I kept secret. Not even Susan knew about this. I didn't want anyone to see me this way, so I usually did this in the middle of the night, in the fortress of solitude that was my room.

Now, it became worse after Susan was gone. I started lying to my parents to get more money for school just so I could buy more food for myself. I used to have one milkshake, a cheese hamburger, French fries, and an ice cream brownie. I ate all of this in about twenty to thirty minutes, and when I got home, I had dinner with my family. Other times I would make the same bowl of popcorn, but I'd use 3 to 4 bags, cheese, crackers, cereal, gummy bears, and candy bars. Some other times, I would have a whole gallon of ice cream to myself. Needless to say. I felt absolutely terrible after these binges. I was out of control, and once I started, I could not stop. Of course, I was terribly ashamed, but I was also extremely full and felt as if my bowels were just about to burst open, and yet, I couldn't help getting to that point.

My mother has always loved me, as I am. She never cared about my weight as long as I was happy, and I tried my best to make her think I wasn't miserable. She already had her hands full with my sisters. My oldest sister was constantly causing trouble at school, so I don't really blame her for being unable to realize I had issues with my weight. My father was mostly too busy at work to realize, and he left most of our upbringing to my mother, so there's no way that he would've been able to realize everything that I was going through if my mother wasn't able to either. And my sisters had their own worries and lives, they were too busy with their own duties and social obligations to go knocking at my door in the middle of the night.

I believe that the first time she found out about this was a couple of months after my Binge-Eating had become worse; when I could no longer fit into my clothes and I had to ask her for a new wardrobe. The scale pointed out that I had gained about 12 pounds, going up to 181 pounds. My eyes were probably watery as a sign of the flood that was going on underneath. She grabbed me, held me with her arms, and told me it was going to be okay. I remember feeling like I didn't really deserve her. She was helping me get through a mess that I'd got myself into with my lack of self-control, but my mother is a beautiful person, and I'm very lucky to have her.

That was clearly another deep blow - the fact that I had to get a new wardrobe only made me feel worse. We had to go shopping. I had to say goodbye to the few pieces of clothing that I actually liked, and my mind could not let go of the fact that I was a fat disgrace, an embarrassment, a land whale - something I wished with all my heart that I wasn't. For those of you who've gone through the experience of getting a new wardrobe because you've gained weight, you know what this feels like. The shame of putting on the new clothes, looking at yourself in the mirror, and realizing how you look, it's excruciating. It shouldn't be a surprise for anyone that I had a huge binge-eating episode that night.

It didn't take too long for my classmates to catch up. They noticed that my clothes changed, and they turned up the heat of the bullying. It got to the point where I would cry in the bathrooms of the school. I was extremely unhappy. Sometimes I would even binge around my tears, wetting crackers and Pringles with their salty and disgusting flavor. Crying to yourself in a public bathroom, not an absolutely private place, knowing very well that at any given moment someone could walk in and hear you like this, that's a pit I wouldn't wish on anyone.

I started to read about diets. I no longer wanted to be overweight; I wished that a genie could just show up and grant me a wish so I could stop being this way. So I started to eat less in my regular meals. I even tried to skip some of them, but by the end of the day, I was so hungry, anxious, and tired that I was assaulted by a new binge-eating episode. I didn't want anyone in my family to know that I was trying to lose weight because it was embarrassing to try to stay on a diet, lose weight, and fail so hard in it. My failure was made evident by everyone around me in school, and quite frankly, every time I saw that reflection in the mirror.

I could no longer hide the way I felt. My mother was already aware of that, so she tried to help me by cooking healthier meals and replacing most of our snacks with more healthy alternatives. Our shopping bags were no longer full of Cheetos and Oreos, and instead, my mother bought different kinds of fruit. Instead of the usual bacon strips, scrambled eggs, and toast for breakfast, my mother gave us oatmeal with a banana. She only meant this new diet to help me lose weight, but she couldn't start giving me a different kind of food than the food she gave the others, so my whole family was stuck with my diet. This made me feel even guiltier because now my mother was trying to make me lose weight on one side while I wasted her efforts with every binge on the other. It made me feel like I was disappointing her. Plus, I felt that now my family had a reason to resent me. They were also stuck with my change of diet, and nobody said anything about it. My sister's lips were sealed, but I didn't think it was fair to them, and I can't imagine they would've felt otherwise.

Just to be fair, my sisters really didn't say anything to me about it. I could feel their resentment. I know that they loved our mother's cooking as much as I did, and now they were forced to eat a toned-down version of it. When we started eating fewer hamburgers and more salads, their discontent was evident. And yet, they never said or did anything to me, even though I was obviously the reason for that change of diet.

Sometimes I felt so bad about myself, so flawed, so unfit, that I wanted to die. I wanted it all to end. This was no way to live; this was so unfair. I just could not control myself. Other times, my sadness and distress were replaced by wrath. I was angry at myself;

I was the one doing this to me after all. I should've been capable of choosing when, how, what, and how much was I eating, just like any other person, but I was not. I was the one to blame, and my misery was all because of me. When I looked at myself in the mirror, I saw my worst enemy. I hated her so much, and for the way that she was treating me, for the things she was making me do, I was sure that the feeling was mutual.

However, I never did feel at risk of committing suicide. I knew that I didn't have the guts to do it, and the thought of my mother kept me from even considering it as a viable alternative. She didn't deserve it. She didn't deserve to get home one day and find out that her daughter was gone, taken away from her so early, and, most of all, in such a terrible way.

But that left me exactly where I was. I still had a huge problem, I was still miserable, and I was still a victim of bullying, and I still hated myself. I was sinking deep in my depression. I was still binge-eating amounts of food that could feed three grown men, and I could not help it. I was out of control.

This kept going until one day; one of my classmates decided that it would be a great idea to spill his yogurt over me in front of the whole cafeteria. He said some awful things about me that I would not write here, but it doesn't matter anyway. The only thing that matters is how bad I felt. I ran out of there while the other kids were making fun of me, and the school called my parents. I had to half-heartedly go back there and sit with them whilst the director lectured my classmate about the politics of the school regarding this kind of behavior. The kid was suspended, but this just made everything worse. I felt even more humiliated because now my parents were involved, now they knew about the awful things that happened to me inside of school. It made me feel like even more of a disappointment.

At the time, I wanted to disappear. I wanted to leave this world so badly that I started picturing ways to do it. I could not see a way out of my misery. I was gaining weight, I hated myself, hated my body, and the things that made me feel that way were growing in me. It was like riding in a train set on fire, a train directed to hell. You know you don't want to be there; you know you want to get out, especially before you get any further because the more you advance, the worse everything gets, but you just don't know how to stop. I couldn't stop my binge-eating episodes. I could feel a death wish growing inside of me, and I wasn't sure that I was able to control that one either.

This is the lowest I had been. I came to weigh 188 pounds. I was utterly disgusted by my own reflection. I could no longer look at my father in the eyes because of the shame I felt. I was tormented by a disease I didn't know I had, and I was my own worst enemy.

This had to change. I had to get serious about that, about getting better. The struggle against my disease was starting to become a life-or-death situation. You know what they say. Once you hit bottom, the only thing left to do is to go up.

Chapter Three

True Change is About the Little Steps

A t that moment, I knew that I couldn't continue to be the way I was. I wasn't healthy, I wasn't normal, and I'd finally realized that it was not a matter of going through a rough couple of months or years. My behavior was inadequate, and I had to do something about it.

Know Your Enemy

The first thing I did was research. I already thought of myself as a depressed person. I had heard that one of the symptoms was an increase in appetite, so that was my first guess.

I started reading webpages, forums, even books in the library. After some research, I was able to understand a couple of things better regarding my mental disease.

I constantly felt sad, had suicidal thoughts, ate way too much, and overslept. I also had a very low image of myself, so I did have some things in common with depression. I didn't know whether it was major depression or something else. I was suffering from something of the sort; after reading about it, it all started to make sense.

Looking into my most relevant symptom, my binges, I ran into Binge-Eating Disorder and Bulimia Nervosa. This was more like my illness, I had an eating disorder, and this completely described the monster living inside of me. I understood that I wasn't a bulimic because I didn't purge. I was unable to control the feeding urges, I couldn't stop eating once I started a binge-eating episode, and most of all, I felt awful afterward. The difference with Bulimia Nervosa was that I didn't vomit, use laxatives, or compensate in any other way after my binges.

I know this may sound insensitive, but it is the truth. I could not help but wish to resemble more the girls suffering from Bulimia Nervosa. Most of them were skinny and beautiful, and I felt it couldn't hurt me to be more like them. Later on, I realized how childish I was to think that way. Either way, the difference was clear. People suffering from Bulimia Nervosa did suffer from Binge-Eating, they were also unable to control their impulses regarding food that they purged afterward, so they maintained their weight (sometimes they even lost it). Of course, Bulimia Nervosa isn't healthy either, vomiting constantly is bad for your digestive system, and it increases the risk of developing cancer, not to mention the way that disease affects your mind. Nobody should ever wish to suffer from that disease.

I found Binge-Eating Disorder. Back then, some people were speaking about it as being separate or its own disorder, completely separated from Bulimia Nervosa. I found this description to fit me best. I was Binge-Eating; I was eating an abnormal amount of food within a small period of time. I was unable to control it. I felt terribly guilty afterward, and full. To this day, I'm not sure how my stomach managed to keep everything in. I made sure to do it when nobody was watching me because I was ashamed of it. I'm sure I didn't do it because I was hungry. I also did it often enough. At first, it was once per week or so, but by my worst period, I was Binge-Eating about twice to three times per week.

So that was it, I had to dig into it because not everyone was talking about this, and not everyone knew what to do about it, but I was sure of it. I suffered from Binge-Eating Disorder, I was sick, and I had to do something about it before the consequences got worse.

First Steps

What I found when I was looking for a solution to my problem was that most people were focused on losing weight. Back then, people with Binge-Eating Disorder were treated just like obese people. They were sent to fat camps (my dad almost forced me to go to one, but thankfully my mother stopped him). They received behavioral weight loss treatment, diet, and exercise. If you're suffering from Binge-Eating Disorder, and you've tried this approach, you'll know that this isn't exactly the best way to treat someone suffering from this disease, but at the time it was what I had, so I decided to give it a go.

I put together a diet plan based on meals that were ridiculously small, and I started an exercise routine based on mild stretches and walking for about 30 to 45 minutes. By the end of the day, I was starving. I was really tired, and I would lose control and start binge-eating.

When my episode was over, I was so ashamed that I used to lie in my bed just looking at the ceiling, avoiding at all costs seeing any part of my disgusting body. The next morning, I made a bigger effort. I tried to eat less, and I tried to exercise more. My anxiety increased. I was always stressed, anxious, and hungry. My binge-eating episodes were getting more aggressive, and I wasn't losing weight, I was gaining it.

And just like that, I had created a negative cycle of self-destruction. I starved myself during the day, then I got home and started with the shameful parade of the dish after dish of embarrassing food. Most times, I got discouraged by my own failure at staying true to my diet, so I started binge-eating immediately after that. If I was by myself in the school and I had one cookie, that threw me off, and I would start telling myself something along the lines of "It's no use now, I've already failed, I might as well go all the way today and have a couple of cheeseburgers on my way home".

This approach was not helping me at all. I still felt inadequate, fat, and mostly embarrassed. I was unable to control myself. If I didn't have the strength to stop myself from binge-eating, what made me think that I could do it along with keeping a diet? Most people fail when they try to follow such rigorous diets. Why would I succeed, considering I already lacked self-control in the first place?

It was delusional to believe that I could do it, and honestly, take this as my advice, don't try to do it either. Trying to follow strong, rigorous diets is one of the biggest mistakes a Binge-Eater can make.

I know that now. I went to my therapist, and both the knowledge and treatments for Binge-Eating Disorder are more advanced nowadays. Nevertheless, if you have tried to do it, or if you're trying to right now, I wish you good luck, but don't beat yourself up too much if you fail. Binge-Eating Disorder should not be treated with regular diets and exercise. The excess weight is not your disease. It's the consequence of it; the treatment should be focused on the disease instead of the consequences.

After a couple of months, and gaining ten pounds, I knew for sure that this was not working. I had read a lot about the importance of getting help from your family and friends. I also knew that if I was going to take this seriously, I should get professional help. I was avoiding this at all costs because I didn't want my family to find out. I was scared to my bones at the way my parents would look at me after that, but I had tried to do it on my own, and it didn't work.

It was time for me to get some help. And I can say that this is as true for me as it would be for every single one of you.

Getting help was the right choice.

Chapter Four

Getting My Family Involved

For those of you that already know that you're suffering from Binge-Eating Disorder and are reading this book to find out what to do about it, this is the first true recommendation that I'm giving you. You should, absolutely, by all means, go to your family for help.

I understand how some of you feel about this. You don't want to get help because you don't want your family to see you like this. You may think that your disease is not serious enough, or they'll definitively see you as a weirdo, a sick person, and you're not there yet. You're still normal, and you don't deserve to be perceived that way. Well, I understand it completely, but that's the wrong way to put it. The truth is that you need help. We all need help. We all need to take Binge-Eating Disorder seriously, and if you believe you're not bad enough that you need to tell your family, I'd still advise you to go right now. You don't want to wait until things are so messed up that there'll be no way around it.

I remember that I was so scared that my hands were sweating. It was dinnertime, and we were all sitting around the table, and I was going over the exact words I intended to use in my mind. "I'm suffering from Binge-Eating Disorder; it is a real disease. I need your help".

My forehead was sticky, and my knees were trembling. I knew that I had to go over this, I needed help, but I didn't want to change the way my family saw me. I'd spent the last week picturing this moment, repeating the possible scenarios over and over in my head, and most of them terrified me. But I took a leap of faith; for my sake, I summoned the courage and did it.

So I was at the dinner table with my family. I took a deep breath, drank a mouthful of water, dried my lips with the napkin, and started talking. "Mom, Dad, I need to tell you something." Once I got my head started, I was able to draw out everything that was on my mind. I stuttered, I paused whenever I needed to gather my thoughts, and I resumed talking when I found the words to continue. To my surprise, they didn't make me feel bad at all. They were just very concerned about my wellbeing. To this day, I'm still very grateful for my parents as they were so supportive they made me wish I had gone to them earlier.

And then my dad said something that gave me chills. "Very well then, you are going to a fat camp. My side of the family has a tendency to being overweight, and I know that won't be good for your health in the future". My father is overweight, but not dangerously so. His brother, on the other hand, is obese, and his father, my grandfather, died from a heart attack, an event related to his weight.

Nevertheless, the idea of going to a fat camp terrified me. I knew what happened at those places. You were forced into huge exercise routines and very strict diets. I already knew what that kind of routine meant for me, and it wasn't good. I started to discuss with him, begging him to understand that I had already tried diet and exercise, and it only made things worse, hoping he would see my problem as it was, a deep lack of self-control. As a sixteen years old teenager, I didn't hold high hopes about this. It's not easy to be taken seriously by your parents when you're that age. If it weren't for my mother, I would have probably ended up gaining more weight in one of those camps.

"You're not taking my baby away, especially if we're not sure that it's the best thing for her. The best thing we could do is to hire a therapist."

And it was settled. My mother had saved me from what would have been a terrible experience. My knees were no longer shaking, my hands were dry, and I was recovering control over my breathing. For those of you who have considered such a place, fat camps are not the best way to help someone with Binge-Eating Disorder. You can't face this problem using hard discipline alone, and suffering in front of a group of strangers will not help either.

Down the road, I found the huge positive power this choice had in my life. My family got involved in my recovery. They helped me keep track of my food and motivated me to follow my diet. The best thing was when I started to get better; they would cheer me on and congratulate me. I could feel their love and support, and it really made a difference, and I feel extremely grateful for it. I understand that some of you may not run with the same luck, but I believe that there's at least someone for every one of you out there. Maybe if you ask someone to help you'll receive a happy surprise.

For me, my family decided to help me with my disease. My therapist, the psychiatrist, ran family therapy with us, and I think that thanks to that, they knew better about how to help me. I was set on the right track to recovery. After therapy, my mother started to cook different meals for us, so that I could eat healthier while my sisters had the liberty to eat pizza for dinner if they wanted to. I understood the way my family felt about me, and my family understood the way I felt. The psychiatrist taught them different ways to support me in my recovery and to avoid harming my feelings. You'll end up wishing you had taken them sooner to the therapist as the change in your life is real; having the support of your family can save you.

Binge-Eating Disorder path is a hard one, and nobody should walk it by themselves. Allow your family to be there for you.

Chapter Five

Serious Help

Dear readers, this is the next true advice I am going to give you. I am positive that every single one of you will deeply benefit from this decision.

You need to get professional help.

It doesn't matter if it's a clinical psychologist, a therapist, or a psychiatrist, although if you want someone who is able to give you medication, you should probably go to a psychiatrist. Therapists and clinical psychologists are not allowed to prescribe medications in California (it changes with the state). Still, whenever a clinical psychologist makes the decision to give you medication, he is able to send you to a physician with a recommendation, so they're the ones doing the prescriptions.

If you're having trouble getting professional help because of some sort of the wrong preconception about it, there's something right there that needs some work. First of all, I want you to think about your mental illness in the same way you'd think about any other illness. You wouldn't think it strange for somebody suffering from a heart attack to go to a physician. That's normal. That's what society expects them to do. Binge-Eating Disorder, just like any other illness, works the same way. If you're sick, you're expected to go to a doctor and try to get healed. People with Binge-Eating Disorder, or any other mental illness for that matter, should be expected to go to a psychiatrist, clinical psychologist, or therapist, and it's no reason to be ashamed.

"I'm not that sick. If I go to a shrink, I'll be like those sick people that are messed up in the head." Well, once again, there's no reason to be embarrassed about that. Suffering from a mental illness is something that just happens. It's not your fault any more than it's your fault if you suffer from a medical condition. It's just something that happens, and as bad as it is, as much as it may affect your personal life, you shouldn't have to go through it without professional help.

Anyway, looking for a therapist wasn't easy. I had made it clear to my father that I wasn't going to go to a fat camp, and that he should take my illness seriously, so we were looking for someone who knew his way around Binge-Eating Disorder. Back then, that was not extremely common.

After doing some research and asking for recommendations, my parents finally took me to a psychiatrist. She specialized in children and teenagers, so she was experienced with eating disorders, and she knew what to do with us. She was a professional, and she knew full well what to do with me and how to deal with my issues. She made me feel safe.

One of the first things she gave me was a new diet plan. To my surprise, this plan had five meals per day, and they weren't all salads either. It even allowed me one snack per day. This all seemed really odd for me, but she was sure that this would work, and I had to trust her, especially after my experience with my own diet.

She also took me to group therapy. Once a month, I would meet with eight other bingers. When I got with them, I felt like we all were looking at the world through the same glasses. We shared problems, most of us looked alike regarding our weight, so I no longer felt alone. It also helped me understand what could go wrong if you don't get treatment. There are more ways in which this disease can affect you than are readily apparent. Living the different effects, this disease could pose a threat to my life though knowing their experiences were good for me. It taught me the value of facing this disease with a serious approach. Binge-Eating Disorder is serious, and it's not to be taken lightly.

Through group therapy and solo therapy, we worked on my personal relationships. My psychiatrist told me that my disease affected the way that I related to everyone around me, the way I saw those relationships, and the way they influenced me. In a way, I ended up having a growing cycle of unhealthy human relationships, both influenced by my disease and influencing it, making it worse.

This didn't happen just with personal relationships. This phenomenon was also present in my thoughts, actions, and my view of the world. If I thought that I was helpless, that made me lose control over my binges, and losing control over my binge-eating episodes made me feel more helpless. We also had to work on that as this was crucial for my recovery, and I know that helping you see these kinds of patterns in your life will help you cope with this illness.

She also gave me a prescription. At first, my father didn't agree with it, but the psychiatrist convinced him that it was the best way to go. She gave me Zoloft, and I feel that it helped me. Being honest, at first, I didn't feel anything. They only caused mild nausea, which certainly wasn't pleasant, but it did somehow reduce my appetite, so I guess there's a silver lining in there. If I stopped taking it, I would feel weird, almost as if I was going down on a rollercoaster, and when I started taking it again, it would hit me harder in my stomach. Nonetheless, whenever I took my pills with discipline, they helped me feel better. It was somehow easier to feel better about myself, less embarrassed about who I was, and I know for sure that it reduced my binge-eating episodes.

Chapter Six

Keeping a Journal

My psychiatrist made it very clear that my illness had more to do with other aspects of my life than food. She told me that she had a good idea of what it was related to, but if I wanted to be sure, I would have to do some deep digging.

So once every week we would meet in her office. We would speak about how things were going at school, at home, and most of all, she let me go on and on about how I felt.

So I talked for hours about how much I hated my classmates, how I missed Susan, and mostly, how much I hated myself for the disaster I'd become. The rest of the days, I didn't see her. I was to keep a journal of everything that I thought was significant about my day. I was supposed to write about these things and how they made me feel. Of course, it goes without saying that I was to document my binge-eating episodes.

I learned that journaling is an excellent way to get to know yourself. It has a way of helping you organize your train of thoughts. Writing about myself forced me to pour my mind over the paper in an orderly manner, and reading my journal allowed me to look at myself in a different way.

For instance, I already knew that I hated my body. I really despised the way I looked in the mirror. What I learned for sure after reading my journal was that if something particular happened that made me over conscious of my body weight, it made me feel worthless, and later on that day, I would probably fall into a binge-eating episode.

If I spent hours on the bed, feeling my body that really messed with my self-esteem. I would think about how my fat was splattered at both sides of myself; I could feel it with my elbows as I laid there holding a book in front of me. I would feel the way my fat thighs touched one another even if I spread my legs, trying not to think about it, and just thinking about my body did horrors for me. To this day, sometimes, it still makes me feel bad.

If by any chance, I looked at myself in the mirror and thought that I had gained some weight, this thought ripped me apart. Sometimes I made a bold choice regarding clothing, and I chose to dress in something reckless. 80% of those times, I would regret it and feel worse. So I mostly wore oversized sweaters and sweatpants in order to hide my body. If anyone did make a remark regarding how I looked, that also made me feel awful. It's one thing to know that you look hideous, but it becomes a whole different matter when you know someone else sees it too.

I was also tempted by some different kinds of food, just like anybody else. Staring at a bag of Oreos, Reese's, or Cheez-It pushed forward the intrusive thoughts in my head. Walking home alone from school and taking a detour close to my favorite diner almost always meant that I was going to wind up eating there. You must look at those things that tempt you, the triggers of your binge-eating episodes, and avoid them at all costs. Before I had my daughters, when I first moved in with Alex, we didn't have any snacks that increased the danger of my binge-eating episodes in the house. We did everything we could to avoid these temptations because I knew that, considering that I was no longer living with my parents and I would spend more time by myself, avoiding the binge-eating episodes would be harder.

There were other patterns to look into; some other things that later on came to make sense thanks to my psychiatrist. For example, those days in which I felt particularly loved by my mother, I was less likely to binge-eat. It was as simple as that. If my mother was particularly nice to me, I would feel much better. That sort of protected me against my disease.

So, having a good relationship with my mother and my family helped me with my disease. I also found the opposite to be true. On those days, when I got in a fight with my family, no matter what it was about, I tended to binge-eat more. Having a good relationship with your family can save you from Binge-Eating Disorder. I feel like this is the first place we should look whenever we're investigating the origin of our mental illness. I can't say that my family is messed up, for that matter, but there's more to us that comes from our environment that we give credit to. We should pay more attention to the way we treat those around us, especially our loved ones.

I know it may sound petty, but I figured that comparing myself to my sisters also did no good. Looking at them after looking at me, being around them as they got attention, and I didn't, all of this messed with my head. If one of them was looking particularly beautiful, it would make me feel like some kind of ogre. I know this sounds stupid, but I couldn't help feeling that way. I could feel the way people stared at me at parties whenever I was with them. Their honest smiles changed to a more awkward facial expression when they turned from my sisters and greeted me. People treat you differently when you don't fit into society's beauty goal, and it shows. You're aware of it even from such a young age.

One of the top triggers for my binge-eating episodes was the bullying I received in the school. It seems fairly obvious. I would bet that as you're reading this, you probably have one thought or two about what triggers your binges, but believe me, it is not the same. It feels different when you're sure they're related when you look straight at a pattern and know that you just found out something about yourself for sure.

So if I heard people laughing behind my back, whenever I felt rejected by my peers at school, especially whenever someone said something nasty to me, I felt horrible, and I would have trouble avoiding binges that night. These interactions with my peers left me with a sour taste in my mouth, and I carried a huge hole in my chest all-day-long afterward. Words have power. People can bring you up and down as easily as turning a switch, especially if you don't have good self-esteem or a strong sense of who you are.

And the food - the food my mother cooked made me feel almost as good as her affection and reassurance. I had what my psychiatrist liked to call an ambivalent relationship with food. One part of me really loved it; the other part of me hated how it made me feel. Food made me feel warm inside while I was eating it, and then I would be really embarrassed when I had finished eating. This is something almost all bingers share. Whenever I read in forums or talk with a fellow binge-eater, I can tell we felt very similarly about food. People say love and hate are just one step away from each other, and I feel like it's true. You can love and hate something at the same time. It's not healthy, whether that happens with someone else, food, or any other important aspect of your life, for that matter.

You must understand what's bothering you. As my psychiatrist taught me, mental diseases are often just a way of coping with our issues - wrong ways, childish ways, often immature, but that's just it. We have to work on ourselves so we can face our issues as healthy people do, and we have to work on our issues in order to recover some of our lives. In order to work on my issues, I needed to recognize them first, to really understand how I felt. This is something that all of you must do.

Sun Tzu said, "If you know neither your enemy nor yourself, you will succumb in every battle." In order to fight against Binge-Eating Disorder, you must know it, get familiarized with your triggers, and what developed the disease.

Chapter Seven

The Sickness Around Me

———————◁◆◁▷◆▷———————

We are, after all, products of our environment. We tend to perceive ourselves the same way as the others see us. We are constantly looking for praise and validation, so it is not hard to believe that the environment plays an important part in the development of Binge-Eating Disorder.

I advise you to study deeply that which makes you feel bad, ashamed, or inadequate. In the previous chapter, we already identified that which makes us feel bad; now, we must look deeply into it, and work to overcome it.

In my case, the earliest starting point of my disease, the first Binge-Eating seed that I could think of was during my childhood. I was overweight long before I started having binge-eating episodes when I was a little girl I didn't binge, but I wasn't a healthy eater either.

As I've already told you, my mother is a great cook, and I've always loved the way she cooks. My mother knew that I liked her cooking, and I think that she felt as if I was the one that appreciated it the most. My mother spoiled me. She has a huge heart, with which she has always loved me very much. In seemed to me that she started building a relationship with me through her cooking. We would laugh together in the kitchen whilst my sisters were out playing in the backyard. I helped her cook our meals. It was a pleasure to watch her work, and she gave me little tastes of her food every now and then. When we were together at the table, I always asked for more after cleaning all the food on my plate, and she would gladly give it to me. In the end, I ate more than I probably should have. Of course, staying in the house cooking and eating didn't do wonders for my figure, so I gained weight until I was fat.

When we got out as a family, my sisters were always so pretty. I didn't feel like I looked so good, and I noticed. I remember clearly one time when one of our uncles was kind enough to say something pretty about each one of us. He told my sisters something about how beautiful they were, and I was left with a bad compliment regarding how I was always smiling. That kind of thing made me feel terrible. It forced me to compare myself to my sisters, to feel like the ugly duckling.

This forged the way I saw myself regarding my sisters, how I related to my family, and how I perceived them. In order to overcome this situation, my psychiatrist helped me understand that I had formed a prejudice regarding this, and it wasn't necessarily the truth. There was no need to compare me to them. Nobody was really doing it more than me, nobody thought of me as the ugly fat sister. It was all in my mind. For those of you who feel that way, I'd tell you that the people who really matter in your life don't compare you, especially in regards to body weight. You're not judged by your appearance by those who love you, even if what they say to you makes it seem that way. When push comes to shove, if you sit them down and talk with them, you'll most likely find that everything that worried you was in your head.

We practiced with the language. We replaced the words with which I thought about them. They would no longer be the thin sisters because that highlighted our difference regarding weight, and it wasn't necessary; no one really cared about that. They weren't the pretty sisters unless I was thinking about the four of us, because being fat doesn't mean I'm not pretty. So instead of thinking about the four of them as the pretty ones while I was some sort of uglier version of them, they all were my sisters, my beloved sisters, and the four of us were the pretty ones. Plus, it was wrong for me to think about them, mostly in terms of how we looked. We were different after all, but if I thought about how we looked different, that made me feel like I was the one that didn't fit, and that happened because I gave too much importance to appearance and bodyweight. If I think of the four of us as complete human beings, we are all different. We have our own personalities, interests, and goals. If you see it that way, we're just different persons. It's not like I'm the fat sister, I'm just another sister; the "fat" label is placed upon me by no one but myself.

It was hard because I actually didn't believe this at first. At first, I would think about them as I always did, and then I would correct myself in my mind. It was like "alright, not the pretty ones, just them," or "she's not the beautiful and thin Andrea, she's just my beloved sister Andrea" (my oldest sister). It was confusing because I always thought of her this way, so a part of me would say back, "but she IS the beautiful and thin Andrea, and I am just the fat and ugly Sophie." After some time, discipline, and treatment, these hurtful thoughts stopped being a sort of burdening natural preconception in my mind, so I didn't think about them that way, and I started feeling better whenever I thought about them.

Changing the way I felt about them was sort of the inside job. In order to overcome this part of me, I had to work on my relationship with them. No longer should I relate with them feeling under. My psychiatrist told me to start treating them as equals, just like sisters, just like we used to play together when we were very, very young. Toddlers don't care that much about bodyweight. Feeling bad about being fat is something they teach us; we're not born this way. There was a time in which we all played together without caring about our weight, height, or how we looked.

Thinking that my sisters were the center of attention also left me feeling as if I would somehow end alone. That is not true, thankfully I'm happily married; but it was something very present in my mind back then, even more than I realized. I didn't know I felt this way; this happened in my mind without me noticing. So I thought that I was going to end alone, and the moment in which I was happiest, when I felt recognized, loved, and praised, was with my mother, especially when we were cooking and eating her food. Food became recognition; it was the love I needed, the thing that saved me from being all alone in this world.

My environment ostracized me because I was fat. I wasn't well-liked because of my weight. I didn't get as much praise as my sisters due to the fact I was overweight. I believe that we, as a society, should think hard about this problem. I don't think that you should be miserable just for being fat. It is alright to want to be thin, to want to look a little bit more like movie stars, but if you don't, this world shouldn't punish you as hard for this. It's only necessary to lose weight when it becomes a health issue, but I wasn't unhealthy when I was a girl. I didn't get to a weight in which I was at risk of suffering from a heart condition until long into my teenage years, and that only happened because of Binge-Eating Disorder. A disease partly caused by the constant torment that I received from my society. So instead of helping fat girls lose weight by giving them a hard time about being fat, you're actually making things worse.

I was afraid I would end up alone. I was sure that this was because of my weight, and at the moment, my classmates were giving me a hard time because of it, and I ended up as an introvert without friends. This truth was made evident for me by the way they treated me. Then I got Susan, and she was a good friend. She was my friend for four years, four years in which I came to grow accustomed to her presence. After that, she left. She was the one that understood me and what I was going through, and she ended up leaving, which hit me hard. I missed her a lot, but I also got really scared, afraid of being alone. After she was gone, I was left without anyone in my life that chose to be related to me.

There was also bullying. My classmates gave me a hard time, a situation that only got worse as I grew older and larger. Their bullying made me feel rejected, and my rejection made me feel worthless. Not only was I alone, helpless, and rejected, I wasn't worthy of love, praise, and recognition. I felt that way about myself, and that belief was reinforced by the bullying I received. My heart is broken, and I can feel the tears rushing towards my eyes as I'm writing these words. Nobody should ever feel this way, especially a teenager, much less when we are talking about a little girl. We need to change. We need to stop this. We are hurting one another, causing harm to people who are very vulnerable and innocent. My environment hurt me, and it ended up in the development of my disease.

Don't get me wrong; I'm not saying that it is all because of your surroundings. Some people are just more vulnerable than others. Stronger people that go through this are able to face these fears without breaking. They are still alone, laughed at, and yet they keep control over their eating habits. Those who suffer from Binge-Eating Disorder are more vulnerable. The disease is born from the marriage of the environment and this vulnerability. I don't intend to make people think that certain environments will surely cause Binge-Eating Disorder; it is just part of the genesis. And for those of us who have it, we must learn to find it in our surroundings in order to defeat it.

Of course, I couldn't just lose weight in order to overcome these issues. Becoming thinner was very hard, I was already working on it, and the results were very slow. Instead of telling me that I would be alright when I started to lose weight, my psychiatrist worked with me on this bias I had about being fat. I was fat. I've been fat all my life, and at the moment, I needed to lose weight mostly for health reasons (I was classified as obese). However, being fat wasn't something to feel so bad about. I needed to lose weight, and I was working on it, but there was no need for me to be as thin as a model in order to be healthy. I wanted to be slimmer, and I gave too much relevance to my bodyweight. It was the cornerstone I used to rate myself and construct my self-esteem. When I started going to therapy, I was considered obese. I needed to lose weight for health reasons, but there was no need for me to lose weight until I got as thin as a model. Once I got to a healthy weight that would be enough. If I wanted to keep getting slimmer, that was alright, too, but I had to be able to be happy with that overweight. We're too focused on raising our self-esteem just as the scale goes lower. We had to work in that mindset that only allows us to feel good about ourselves if we're slim.

It's readily apparent that being overweight didn't mean that I was going to die alone. My psychiatrist started working with me on the way I thought about myself. In this case, it was subconscious, so we worked with positive reinforcements. She would have me repeat over and over in my head that there were people in this world that loved me, so I would also say it out loud when I was alone in my room I also wrote it down in a notebook over and over again. At first, it felt really silly, but I got used to it. Positive reinforcement helped me feel better on a level in which I wasn't able to work directly. The effects of this therapy happen at a subconscious level, so you should give it a try even if you don't think it's useful. Keep in mind that this isn't my recommendation alone, my psychiatrist and many other therapists think the same way. You should think about that before tossing positive reinforcements aside.

We also worked on my personal relationships. As it turns out, believing that people didn't want to have anything to do with me made me more distant, sort of pushing people away from me. I started to get in touch with Susan. She was doing fine in her new school, making new friends, and missing me as much as I missed her. To this day, Susan is still my friend. We've managed to stay in touch after all these years. Sometimes, all you have to do is reach out to those you care for. In my case, I had Susan. She was no longer around, but we could still call and text each other, and that made a difference in my mood.

I also started to work on my relationship with my family. I was already close to my mother, but I tried to get closer to my father and my sisters. I was very glad to find that all I needed was reaching out. I asked my father to teach me music, and he gladly set aside some free time to teach me how to play the piano. I was terrible, but it was a great way to get closer to him and to keep my mind occupied. Word of advice, getting a hobby is also helpful. It was good for me to stop thinking about everything that was troubling me; plus, when I started to get better, the sense of fulfillment made me proud of myself. My psychiatrist told me that it was going to help me a lot with my self-esteem, and she was right. I kept my journal, and I found that on those days on which I practiced with my father, I was less likely to binge-eat. It's amazing how these little things have the power to impact your life. In the end, the disease is just as a manifestation of your life not being in order. Putting your life together is the best solution.

When I started to get closer to my sisters, I found that they were happy to go out with me. I didn't do it enough back then because I was just full of self-embarrassment. I didn't want to go out and have people stare at me. But after talking to my psychiatrist, I understood that it was something I needed, and she was right. Besides, people at the school were mean, but people on the street actually do not care if you are fat. After some treatment, working on my train of thoughts, and trying to reprogram my mind, I understood that most of the impolite stares at me were in my mind.

So we started going out. I started to socialize with their friends, and I felt like I fitted in. Being all alone because I was fat was a boundary that I had placed over myself, the reality was different. People were able to accept me for who I was, so there was no need for me to be alone.

The school was a whole different matter. Kids tend to be really mean, and if they've been mean to you your whole life, it is hard to get them to like you. In the end, my psychiatrist recommended a transfer to another institution. After everything that happened to me at school, it wasn't hard to convince my parents to do it. Considering that the strongest negative impact on my life came from my school, a change of scenery did wonders for me. Of course, I was a new girl. I wasn't exactly popular. Even though I tried, I was still an introvert, so I didn't make friends on the first day, so to speak. Still, I wasn't bullied anymore, so the biggest stimulus that produced binges in my life was gone. Plus, after I was transferred, I got to meet Alex, my husband; thanks to that, my two beautiful daughters were born. That transfer changed my life for the better.

Knowing yourself is the true battle with the biggest rewards. Binge-Eating Disorder has a lot to do with your environment. Some people claim that you must first change yourself in order to change the environment; others ask for a better environment just to be better. The truth is that you should never depend on the environment, but getting better when you are swimming in a toxic pool is almost impossible. The important thing is to take action. You can't expect your surroundings to get better; you must do it yourself. And you can't wait until you're better before you start working in your environment. You must start working right away; it's the only way. This is something that every single one of you must focus on in order to heal, and now you have the tools to do it.

Getting out of that toxic pool and catching fresh air feels amazing. You still have internal issues to work on, but now it's like you don't have the whole world against you. Of course, receiving some toxicity is inevitable, but it is never the same, and now you have a way to shield yourself from it.

Chapter Eight

Middle Ground

I was absolutely right when I told my parents that I didn't want to go to a fat camp.

Those places may work for oversized people without Binge-Eating Disorder, but they would have been awful for me. Following a strict and oppressive diet with lots of exercises is not the best strategy for someone suffering from Binge-Eating Disorder. If you have attempted to do this and failed, don't feel bad about it. It's actually pretty hard for us to follow these kinds of plans.

The fact is that if you don't have the discipline if your will is weak if you lack self-control, and if your mind is working against you, this will be counterproductive. This is especially the case since you're going to end up on a binge-eating episode because you're feeling terrible after your failure. We're quick to think of ourselves that way. A minor slip is enough to feel like a failure, like a shameful waste of space, unworthy of the effort of getting better.

So, let me show you what this looked like for me when I started the diet. I looked through magazines about slim diets. After the research, I tried with one or two portions of fruit for breakfast, a salad, vegetable soup and a fruit shake for lunch, and a dinner that consisted of chicken breasts, vegetables, and (not too much) rice. I could have a slice of whole bread to go with that breakfast, but it was stretching it. If I had to eat a different breakfast in my home, something heavier, I would try to compensate by skipping lunch. Snacks were absolutely forbidden. I wasn't allowed to eat Pringles, popcorn, ice cream, peanut butter, and jelly sandwiches, none of it.

Dieting didn't seem enough for me at that time. I also wanted to exercise in order to really lose that weight. I started to walk around the neighborhood for about 30 minutes per day. I wanted to jog, but I didn't trust my knees to keep up with my weight just yet. Sometimes I rode a bicycle around, that was more fun, but it was also a lot harder. After some time, I started to feel dizzy if I tried to exercise after eating like a baby. Sometimes I felt like I could've passed out over my bicycle. This didn't allow me to get going, so I ended up going back home earlier than I intended. Going back without having done a complete workout filled me with shame.

The first day I was really proud of myself. I managed to keep my diet. I was absolutely starving, but I was proud. The next day my stomach was making noises that should've been able to wake up my sister in the next room. I was starving; a banana, a slice of watermelon, and a toast with coffee weren't enough for me. I swear that I looked at my food, and I could smell the scent of bacon that I longed for.

I headed for school with my lunch prepared in my backpack, but I took a detour before going to class so I could buy a candy bar from a vending machine. I was so hungry; I thought that I was about to pass out. I was in danger of eating my notebook. After finishing my candy bar, I felt extremely guilty. I was ashamed, fully disgusted by myself. Everything that I had worked for was gone in a matter of seconds, and this was just the second day.

Maybe a normal, overweight person would've left it at that. She would have gone to her class, eaten her lunch, and tried to recover and keep on with the diet. This was not the case for me; I just felt awful for the rest of the day. I didn't have lunch. A part of me thought it was because I was just trying to lose what I gained with that candy bar. But, another part of me deep down knew that I was weak. Skipping lunch wasn't an issue because I would have a binge-eating episode later.

And so I did. I headed to my favorite dinner as soon as I got out of school. I ordered two cheeseburgers, a large portion of French fries, a milkshake and a chocolate brownie. Afterward, I just went home. I was unable to look at myself in the mirror, and I had a normal out-of-diet dinner with my family. That day was already a loss.

This is the way it went for me during that period of time. You know the rest; it didn't help me at all. I ended up gaining pounds, with wider hips and a larger belly. It was awful, as awful as it would've been in a fat camp.

The thing about binge-eaters is that we tend to think only in extremes. We're either doing amazing or doing terrible. We're having success, or we're a total failure. We're either trying the best we've got, or we've lost everything, and it makes no sense to go on. When you feel like that, any mistake will crush your plans for the day. You just don't see the point to keep trying after you've failed. This is not something that happens only with food. Right now, I'm jogging in my spare time to try to lose weight. I'll try to jog for at least 20 or 30 minutes non-stop, but get this, if I stop, even if it's just for a second, it stops making sense to me because I've already failed. At that point, I call it a day, and I go back home.

This mindset doesn't allow us to lose weight properly using classic weight-loss techniques. So forget about strict diets, chances are that they are going to hurt you more than helping you. My psychiatrist worked a diet plan with me that I was able to follow through, and it was a lot easier than that. We often try diets and fail because we perceive them as a sort of punishment. We also look at them as something that has to be done for a limited period of time, and then we can forget about it. Both are wrong and lead to failure.

What we really need to do is eat normally. My psychiatrist wanted me to have pancakes, just no more than two or three of them. I could have Subway, steak, mashed potatoes, and whatever else I wanted for lunch. Then, in the night, I had a normal dinner with my family. I also ate something in the middle of the morning between breakfast and lunch, and something else between lunch and dinner. These two extra meals were something like fruit, crackers, seeds, or yogurt, something light. I had five meals per day, and if I had a really rough day, I was even allowed a snack. I had something like a candy bar whenever I was having a rough day.

I still had to avoid some kind of meal. I couldn't drink soda, and I was encouraged to pass on everything that was fried, especially meals like bacon. This was still reasonable. After eating a turkey sandwich with mayonnaise, mustard, tomato, and lettuce, with mashed potatoes on a side and grape juice to go with it, I didn't really need to top it all with bacon.

A diet plan can't be too harsh, or we will fail. And we can't feel like we're failing, or we will probably top our failure with a binge-eating episode. I still lost weight with this diet plan because I didn't binge so much. This was also because of my treatment, but a diet plan that didn't make me feel like a disgusting failure every time I tried to follow it and failed was a great help.

I know that you all want to lose weight fast. You want to hit the end of the year, looking like a movie star. You're hoping to lose so much weight during spring break that you'll dazzle everyone when you go back to school.

Sadly, that is not for us. We can't lose weight that fast. We are sick. Binge-Eating Disorder is waiting for us to slip so he can take over and ruin everything for us. Every single step we take must be safe. We must check the floor, stay put, and then move on to the next step. We're very vulnerable and fragile, so we have to be extra careful. I know it may seem unfair to have it harder than everyone else, but that's just how it is. We are special. That doesn't mean that we can't do it, it just means that it will be more amazing when we do.

Finding the middle ground is about going out of the reckless lifestyle we used to have, on the one hand, but avoiding rough and harsh diet plans on the other. We must find the balance to a point where it doesn't feel impossible for us, where the diet plan doesn't feel like a punishment for being us. We actually should avoid the word diet at all costs. My psychiatrist told me to avoid thinking about this as a diet. It was forbidden to me. That word has such a negative aura that it's instantly rejected. I didn't think about it as a diet; neither did I think about it as something with time limitation.

The key to finding this middle ground is to stop thinking of it as a diet and trying to see it as our new, healthier lifestyle. Eating five meals per day is actually what we all should do. In the long run, it helped me to eat less on major meals.

Welcome to your new healthier lifestyle. Get comfortable; you're going to stay here for a long time.

Chapter Nine

Turning Things Around

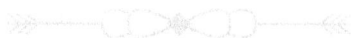

Very well, so now we know how to keep a journal and practice introspection; and the importance that has regarding the recovery of Binge-Eating Disorder. We also know how to work on our environment and our deep relationships. And finally, we know what to do regarding food.

These are the main things we can do to put our life in order and make peace with food. In this chapter, I'll give you some ideas of what to do in order to achieve a better life. Being happy is truly the best defense against Binge-Eating Disorder.

Be More Loving

For me, food was the love that I needed in order to avoid loneliness. I loved and hated it. I ate it just so that I could regret doing it. I needed to work on the relationships I had manner. If the Beatles were right, all that you need is love. I found that the best way to get love is to give it first.

I started every morning by showing affection to my mother. I would hug her, help her with breakfast, and prepare the coffee. Then, I would take a cup of coffee to my father with a kiss on the cheek. I would also try to compliment my sisters if I had the opportunity. I did all of this before going to school. I tried to make more small talk during dinner. I showed interest in them and everything they had to say. Love is often contemplation; all you need to do is to pay attention.

After a while, my father started to smile at me more. We spent more time together. He was full of joy when he was teaching me how to play the piano. I had more quality time with my sisters, to the point in which we started going out together with their friends. Even my mother seemed happier to see me, and I thought she couldn't be more affectionate with me. I also didn't miss the chance to pet animals whenever I could. People that love animals are always surrounded by affection. Dogs are usually very grateful for your love and attention; plus, they return it right away! It's hard to feel grim when you're having your face licked by a puppy.

Being a loving person is a part of my life right now. I try to show my love to my daughters as often as possible, and they return it to me. I love my husband, and he loves me too. We spend time together as a couple and a family. I try to visit my parents every now and then. They love seeing their granddaughters, and we love spending time together as we used to. I also enjoy going out for a cup of coffee with my sisters. We're all busy right now. We can't spend time together like we used to, but once or twice per month, we're able to see each other and catch up.

I don't know for sure if love really is all you need to be happy, but it does get you a long way.

Stay Positive

Positive reinforcement is also an important part of improving your life. I had my room covered with post-it notes that displayed nice messages. Things such as "You're perfect," "You're strong," and "you're in control of everything" were everywhere. This may sound cheesy, and I know that there's a big sector of the population that believes this self-help methodology is nonsense. Nonetheless, I did it, and it worked for me, so I'm placing this here.

Do you know that feeling when you've received a compliment from a member of your family and a part of you is like "alright, thank you, but I know you only say this because you're my family"? I believe you do. My self-esteem issues go way back. I have never been able to trust or properly receive a compliment. If you're suffering from Binge-Eating Disorder, the chances are that you know this feeling too. You may be incredulous, but a part of you deep down still feels warm and fuzzy. Something similar happened to me with the post-it notes I placed all over my room. I read them; I couldn't believe them because I knew that I had written them, and why, and still I felt good inside, even if it was just a tiny bit.

After a while of reading these messages, I started to say these positive things about myself by default in my head. My mind would tell me those phrases that I'd placed on my wall. So if I was, for example, walking home from school, my mind would tell me, "you've got this." It felt great. I was also careful not to go into compliments that specifically regarded my body or my weight. As I'll explain in the next chapter, we must change the mindset of measuring ourselves in terms of beauty and weight. Besides, it was easier for me to believe a compliment about how strong, brave, and clever I am, than to believe that I was stunning, and my body was beautiful. I despised my own body way too much for that.

My mother realized this, and she started to do it too. She was usually very affectionate, but now she started to make positive remarks about me sometimes when we were alone. I knew that she was only doing it to help me, but as I said, it still made me feel warm inside. It didn't take me more than a couple of months to embed these thoughts into my mental system. I still didn't believe them, but my mind used these phrases in me often without making a mental effort. If I'm having a rough day, a part of me, the part that's damaged by the disease, starts to harm me with the intrusive thoughts. Now I am able to immediately start answering, "No, I'm not useless, I'm strong, I'm strong, I'm strong" over and over again.

Fighting against mental illness by being positive may sound silly. Most people won't be even up to try. That is alright. Having someone tell you, "Hey, keep your chin off your chest and stop being sad" when you're depressed is really annoying. It just doesn't work. When you're struggling with mental illness, you can't just put on a happy face and get it over with. I'm not saying that being positive is the way to save yourself from Binge-Eating Disorder. Good and bad moods are not switches that you can turn on and off; however, you please. I'm just stating that surrounding yourself with positive reinforcement is just something else that's able to improve your mood and the way that you feel about yourself. This advice, as well as many other gems from this book, came from my psychiatrist in the form of therapy. We can't just rule it out because it seems naive.

This is just another tool at your disposal. Maybe it's not for everyone, but it's worth the shot.

Find New Sources of Gratification

I've read that people who want to stop smoking often switch that habit for something else. They try to keep their hands busy by flipping coins, working on a Rubik Cube, solving crosswords, eating snacks, etc. Obviously, I can't avoid binge-eating by replacing it with snacks. I must find something else to do in order to avoid binge-eating.

It's a simple concept. You need to find new ways to bring joy into your life if you mean to stop the binge-eating episodes. If food is the only thing that brings you joy, you're in a very bad situation. Binge-Eating Disorder is holding your happiness as a hostage. If you wish to feel it again, you must go dangerously close to it, have a taste of the food you love, and most likely fall into its trap.

I bet that you don't want the disease to have that kind of power over you. In order to take that power away from Binge-Eating Disorder, you must find new ways to bring joy and happiness into your life. Those people who are addicted to cigarettes have it harder because their bodies have developed a chemical addiction to nicotine. In our case, our bodies don't crave food the same way a smoker craves a pack of Marlboro. Switching to a healthier way to find happiness is easier for us.

I've already told you, in this chapter, nonetheless, about the wonders of loving and being loved. Love is the definitive universal way to bring joy into your life. Nothing makes me happier than my family. Watching a movie in the living room, sitting on the couch with Alex with his arms around me, with our daughters in their chairs moving around the floor, is so perfect that I don't even mind they have popcorn in front of me. I have everything that I need right there, the love of my family.

Hobbies are obviously the best way to find joy and fight boredom. During the time I spend alone, I usually take the piano for a spin. It's very easy to download a new chart and start working on it. I'm not a professional pianist. I can't play the most complex pieces from Bach or Mozart, but I can spend a couple of hours learning how to play Let It Go from that Disney movie, Frozen. It's simple, fun, and it's great for singing along at parties or with my daughters.

My husband, for example, spends a lot of time playing videogames. Sometimes I come to watch him play, just to spend some time with him, and he seems to really get lost in it. My daughters, on the other hand, love spending time on Netflix. This one may be dangerous for some of you considering that watching a movie or a TV show is almost an open invitation for a snack; so I guess that unless you're really into it, you should be careful with this one and binges. This is especially the case if you've identified Netflix as a trigger for your binge-eating episodes.

Considering our eternal quest for losing weight, getting a hobby that also allows you to exercise is great for us. I try to make my jogging sessions as fun as I can. I put on my earphones, listen to my favorite music, and sometimes I sing along just for the fun of it. I've never been a fan of sports, but for some of you, finding a sport that you enjoy should be able to bring you joy and help you maintain your figure at the same time. Alex likes to play paintball. He plays in very big fields that demand him to run a lot, so it's a great exercise. He's usually very tired after each session. My daughters like swimming and dancing. They enjoy both activities, and they're both very demanding, so it's a great exercise for them.

Whatever you choose to do in order to bring joy, you should validate it with your journaling. Keep notes of your progress after you start this new activity. If you find that it's helping you avoid the binge-eating episodes, then it is working, and you should stick with that. Of course, a rather healthy option, if possible, is much better. You obviously shouldn't trade food for cigarettes, or alcohol, or any other drug for that matter. You can't go the opposite way either and get a hobby that's so healthy and productive that you don't enjoy it at all. Learning Russian is probably very good for you, but if it's not bringing you joy, you probably should classify it as a self-improvement/work-related activity, rather than a hobby intended to bring you happiness.

Chapter Ten

Improving Your Mental Health

The reason why we have Binge-Eating Disorder is that our minds are a mess. In order to improve, we need to put things in order inside the mind. When you think about fixing your mind, you probably believe it has to do with meditating, and that could actually help you, but that's not what I mean right now. I'm talking about some changes that you must make. These are changes in your exterior, as well as your interior. If you focus on these things, tackling them one by one, I'm positive that you will feel the change. Some of them may seem hard at first, but once you're used to it, you'll them easier to follow than it seems. In this chapter, unlike the previous one, we'll talk about things that are bringing you down right now and how to stop them from doing this to you.

Become a Friend of Your Disease

Binge-Eating Disorder is full of intrusive thoughts that will ultimately tear you down until there is no will left to fight it.

When you're out with your friends, as it occurred to me when I was in the mall with my sisters and their friends, eating in a restaurant may be tricky. If you're already trying to abide by a diet plan, you will probably order a rather healthy option. I would order Chinese food, for example. They have many healthy options, good food, and low prices, so my budget doesn't take a huge blow every time I go order a take-out.

So, you're sitting at the table. You start taking sips of your iced tea, or you take a small bite at your chicken breast or your salad, and then you look around. You see people having pizza, cheeseburgers, and probably a whole bunch of fries. This may be a deep blow for you. You would rather have any of these highly desirable and unhealthy dishes, so the disease kicks in and starts bothering you. "Sophie, you should have ordered that. Look at that peanut butter milkshake, it looks great". You fight it with "No, I can't, you know I can't, stop bothering me." The disease is clever, so it will probably go with "Come on, you know you want to, ask for a sip, just a taste, it won't do any harm," hiding the real meaning of that taste, making it seem harmless. Once you fall, it will hit you as hard as it can with "Now you've done it, it doesn't matter now. You're already a failure; you might as well get one for yourself. Do order some fries with that, they look good".

The disease knows you better than you know yourself because it's right there, in your subconscious. It's familiar with your thought process, the inside workings of your mind. It knows right where your weak points lay, and it's a master at exploiting them.

But after a while, you may become aware of this. You know that stepping just a little bit out of line will do for you. You can feel the feeling of shame and failure building up inside of you as you consider asking for a slice of pizza, so you fight it. You start a long discussion with Binge-Eating Disorder in your mind whilst the rest are busy enjoying their meals. "No, I don't want to eat that. I won't, leave me alone" - "Yeah you do, just look at what you're eating. Perhaps that amount of food was enough for you when you were five years old, but now it won't cut it. You need more, or you'll never be full". I know I've had these conversations, and for what I've researched, for what I learned by interacting with other binge-eaters in group therapy, I'm not the only one with these kinds of thoughts. I guess that you know what this feels like.

Fighting this is losing the battle. This is what I learned. There's no way to take your mind off these thoughts if you keep fighting. You must try to get along with your disease, to calm it down without direct confrontation. Only then you'll have a chance of banishing these thoughts from your mind. If you think about it, it makes perfect sense. There's no way that you can stop thinking about the food if you're leading a discussion with Binge-Eating Disorder about it. All that you will have in your mind is, "No, I don't want to eat it. I don't want to eat it. That food is not good for me. If I drink that, my whole diet will go to waste", and so on.

So, here's what you do. You have to get along to Binge-Eating Disorder. You must be able to negotiate with it instead of fighting it. When it comes to you saying, "Hey, earlier I saw you looking at that bag of Cheetos. I know you want them, quit playing hard, and go have them. It will be so sweet" you must find a way to turn it down politely and offer something else instead. "Yes, Cheetos sounds amazing, but we already had a great lunch. Mom is making spaghetti and meatballs for later, so I want to save my appetite for that". "But the Cheetos are right there; you don't have to wait for dinner," "Yes, but we also love spaghetti and meatballs, and I want to be able to really enjoy them. This will be impossible if we go on and eat that bag of Cheetos all by myself".

After all, the disease is a part of you. You must be able to speak its own language, tear down its desires, and offer something instead that will satisfy it without crashing your diet. This is why it's so important to allow yourself a snack in your diet plan. On the toughest days, it will be easier to calm down the beast if you tell it "Alright, we're having a snack, but it won't be the bag of Doritos XL that you've laid your eyes upon. A strawberry pop-tart will have to do".

This is not as destructive as failing completely. By the end, calming the intrusive thoughts is what matters the most. Binge-Eating Disorder seems like an ugly troll trying to tear you down at first. It's a part of you that you hate, which is pretty easy since your self-esteem is on the ground. But in the end, it is just a part of you. As you come to love and accept yourself, you must be at peace with the disease.

It's going to be with you for a very long time. You might as well get along with it.

Lose the Scale

This one seems absurd, but I found it is in your best interest to stop obsessing about your weight, the measurements of your body, and how you look in the mirror.

Part of my Binge-Eating Disorder was worrying about my food. I was obsessed with it. I wanted to lose weight every day. Every single day I would measure my waist, my arms, and my thighs. It wasn't healthy. If I didn't like what I had, I blamed it on whatever I ate the day before. I felt guilty, and I felt like a failure. Being constantly reminded that you're overweight by your mirror isn't exactly the best way to live and to overcome your issues, especially since it's a gateway for the intrusive thoughts, always ready to take over and ruin your mood.

I understood, at some point, that I needed to take my mind of this. I'm a human being, and as such, I can't be valued just by my body fat percentage. I know this happens because we're used to it. The world taught us that you're valued for your looks. That is linked to your weight. This is especially bad for girls and women. The fashion industry will show you bodies that are very hard to get for most of us. This sets a dangerously hard standard for the way that girls should look, which is a very important factor in the development of an eating disorder.

By all means, we must break this cycle. It's alright to have plus-size models and all of that, but I believe that the problem is still there because we're still valued for our looks. If you're a thin model, you're a model, and if you're a fat model, you're still a top model that's appreciated because of the way you look. This is sad because not all bodies look the same, and that doesn't mean that they're not beautiful. And if your body is not beautiful, that shouldn't be such a big deal. We just care way too much about beauty.

I may be typing these words, and I know they're true, but I also know that they make me a hypocrite. I care about looks. I care way too much, so much that it hurts. I'm embarrassed by my own body. I still don't like it, and if I spend too much time looking at my naked body in the mirror, sometimes, it feels like I might get a panic attack. I still believe that this is no way to live. I fought against it, and I fought it the best way that I could think of.

I'm done measuring me. I've had enough of putting numbers over my body. The inches of my waist, the pounds on the scale, the thickness of my arms and thighs, this is something that I used to measure almost two or three times each week. In regards to my bodyweight, I used to measure it daily. I didn't know how much that hurt me until I let it go. I stopped doing that, and I was able to reduce the intrusive thoughts.

I know what you must think, easier said than done. I understand how you feel. After spending your whole life looking at numbers on a scale and appraising your body in the mirror, it seems impossible just to stop. And you're right; it's not that easy. I'll show you how to do it, but it takes discipline and work.

First, you must literally stop going over to the scale. It may help to throw it out if you need to. You're good as long as you don't measure your weight every single day. This doesn't mean that you'll spend the rest of your life without knowing how much you weight. For medical reasons, and in order to track your progress, you need to. But that doesn't need to happen every single day. My advice is to measure your weight monthly, write it down in a piece of paper you'll have hidden somewhere safe, and then forget about it. Since you have it on paper, your mind doesn't need to remember it; so it becomes easier to forget how much you weigh.

My life is much better since I've stopped thinking about the numbers on the scale. It's just a huge weight off my shoulders. You'll be surprised by how much lighter you feel in your head after you let this worry go. In the beginning, it won't work. It may even get worse since you won't be measuring yourself every day. Your mind might start to do crazy estimations about how much pounds would the scale show you if you were to step over it right now. I know it because that's what happened to me, but luckily I was able to endure that phase I'm much better now. Be aware, since the holiday season is usually bad for our weight, perhaps you'll want to skip the scale in January so that you don't find out how much you gained in December. This could also apply to any difficult period of time in which you binge-eat frequently.

Avoid mirrors at all costs. I used to spend 5 to 10 minutes in front of the mirror after taking a bath, just looking at my body. I felt utterly displeased y the way I looked It was disgusting, and just looking at it was very bad for my mood. The longer I looked, the uglier I felt. I wanted to carve at it with a knife to take away all the things I didn't like, to stop being so flawed, so full of defects. The time I spent in front of the mirror seemed like an eternity; it was awful. After I understood the damage that looking at my body did to me, I knew I had to stop. I couldn't throw away the mirror because my husband uses it to shave, but we got a much smaller mirror and placed it in the bathroom. We gave the bigger one to our daughters, who seem to be very happy playing in front of it. I also try to avoid looking at pictures of myself. If I must, I just try not to stare too long. I know that my eyes will start finding defects in my body, the longer I stare, and I don't want to go through that. Not being as aware of my own body has been good for me. I know I'm overweight. I can look at my arms. I can feel it as I walk. When my husband takes me in his arms and feels my body, I can feel it too. I just can't help it, but I can diminish the self-awareness. As I said, avoid mirrors if you want to keep the troubled thoughts away.

Changing your mindset to worry less about your body is possible. I've spent most of my life being excruciatingly aware of my body weight, but life can be better. I know it is for me right now. We give way too much attention to these things. Quite frankly, as long as you're healthy, you shouldn't have to worry about your weight. The obsession with slimness as the only form of beauty is a disease well spread through our society, and it's making us sick. That's the main reason why we have eating disorders. That's our main problem, and the solution is to stop obsessing about it. The only way for this to harm you is if you let it into your mind. I know it may seem unfair to put it that way because you can't control the intrusive thoughts. They just come to you. Sometimes it's only a drop or two, but sometimes it seems like it's pouring, with thunders rumbling on the background. This may often be the case, I know it was my case, but I was able to achieve it, and I've shown you how I did it, so you should be able to follow my lead.

Throw away your scale or get it somewhere hard to reach so you don't have the temptation to step on it. Do it right now. Put this book down, get to your scale, and do it!

Boredom Is Your Enemy

An idle mind is fertile soil for intrusive thoughts.

I feel that when I started to binge, it had a tendency to happen when I was bored. I had nothing to do, so I opened a bag of peanuts to kill time. Boredom is very common in children and teenagers. It's a disease for the unoccupied. Adults are usually very busy, so most of us don't have the time to get bored, but teenagers do. That's when most eating disorders take place, and most binge-eaters are born. Perhaps that's not a coincidence.

Learning to play the piano wasn't just to get closer to my father. It was also a strategy to fight boredom. When I was focused, especially when I was enjoying myself, I found that intrusive thoughts were not as common. They hit me mostly at night when I was alone in my room; also, when I was walking home from school, vulnerable to taking a detour that might end with a cheeseburger frenzy.

My advice to you is to get a hobby. In my case, playing the piano did wonder for me. I also love to read, but considering that I used to binge-eat whilst reading in my room, using that as a shield against the disease wasn't effective because my mind had them related anyway. A hobby will save you from boredom, and it will keep your mind occupied, leaving no room for the intrusive thoughts.

My work is also very helpful because it demands my whole attention. For all of you out there who work with children, you know how mentally demanding it may be. I have to keep control of my whole classroom, go through my class, and make sure that everyone is paying attention.

It's also something that I really enjoy, so it's easy to get lost into it. Some of you may not be as lucky. You work on jobs that don't require a lot of your attention. You don't love it, so you're often bored while you do it. I've read that truckers often binge-eat on the road, eating huge bags of chips as if they were nothing.

Boring activities, such as studying, are also full of danger. Sadly, sometimes you can't avoid them. The school system often makes you study themes that don't really interest you, so it's a time in which you're often vulnerable to binge-eating. In this regard, my advice is to pursue something that you really enjoy for a living. Studying is not so boring when you're studying something that you really care about. The same goes for work. If you feel like working, if you're eager to go to work, and if you're enjoying yourself during your work shift, you'll most likely be entertained. This is something that probably applies to everyone. Everyone should be working with something they're passionate about.

Fighting boredom may seem hard, but right now, the technology allows us to reach so much information that it's almost possible to do something related to your interests at any given time.

Boredom is another battlefield that we must conquer, and we have the tools and weapons to do it.

Avoid Social Media

We spend way too much time on Facebook, Twitter, and Instagram. It's bad for us as grown professionals because we tend to leave aside our duties to answer the notifications from our phones. Besides, more relevant for this book, it's bad for our mental health.

People don't usually share their whole lives on social media. You won't see somebody's ugly moments on Instagram or Facebook. People choose very carefully what to upload and what not to, as a result, we see the best version of anyone's life on Facebook and Instagram. After we see their perfect pictures, we go through the worst part of our relationship with social media, comparing ourselves with them. It's not fair to compare our everyday version of ourselves to someone else's best version of themselves. That's not a fair competition, and we end up with more pain and mental strain as a result of these comparisons. This isn't healthy for anyone, not just people with Binge-Eating Disorders. You'll find many people on YouTube and their blogs speaking about the benefits of abandoning social media for our mental health. Facebook and Twitter are relatively, very new. We managed to survive without it up until this point, and I'm positive that nobody has lost a limb over erasing their Facebook account. Alright, maybe leaving Facebook entirely isn't necessary. After all, it's the best way to keep up with your relatives; but you should spend less time on it.

First of all, you should erase Facebook's app from your cellphone. It's better for your cellphone and for your mental health. By the end of the day, you'll have more battery. Your days will get to be more productive (not to mention that your personal information will be safer), and you'll likely be in a better mood. Facebook's notifications are the main reason we go in there. Our phones are constantly telling us to go online and check everyone else's pictures. Once you've erased the app, you won't be constantly tempted to go inside. Regarding your desktop or laptop, disable the notifications from Facebook on your web browser.

Instagram is just the same. It might be even worse for your mental health because people have a tendency to play model on Instagram. When you scroll down, you find picture after picture that looks right out of a professional photo shoot; then, you accidentally turn on your camera and see at your face staring right back at you on the screen. I know you've gone through this too. It's unpleasant, unflattering, and awful for your self-esteem. The solution is very simple. Maybe don't erase the app, after all the phone is the best way to access it, just disable the notifications. For me, this was enough; this way, I didn't get a notification every time somebody uploaded a new photograph.

If you have my age right now, or you're older, this step won't be so hard for you. But if you're younger, it will probably be harder for you to get away from social media. Most kids and teenagers nowadays spend most of their time with their noses staring at the screen of their cellphones. They're way too used to this. Turning off the Wi-Fi and taking away their cellphones is an effective way to ground my daughters when they misbehave. It's like hell for them. If you're a teenager reading this book with self-esteem issues and you're going through Binge-Eating Disorder, you probably should spend less time on social media. It's not good for your self-esteem to compare yourself with others 24/7.

Fighting a Binge-Eating Episode

Some claim that there's an effective way to stop a binge-eating episode before it happens. I'm not talking about erasing them from your life, after all, that's more or less the main theme of this book. Up until now, I've spoken to you about how to live in a way that will reduce the binge-eating episodes. Now, let's go over some tips that might stop them cold.

First of all, after all the deep digging you've done, you probably know what triggers most of your binge-eating episodes. Whether if it's boredom, having a bad day, feeling judged, inadequate, or just anxious, you understand what's going on in your life that has the power to summon the horror from the deep. Since you've learned what triggers your episodes, you must be able to tell when you're likely to binge-eat before it happens, even before you start feeling the urge to do it. For example, if I know that spending too much time in front of a mirror is terrible for me if by any chance I happen to run into a mirror in an elevator, and I can't avoid staring, I already know that later on that day I'll be in danger of binge-eating.

You already know how to predict when you'll be binge-eating later. Now, you should be able to feel the urge when it starts to grow inside of you. If you're already aware that you've gone through a trigger that's likely to make you fall into a binge-eating episode, it shouldn't be hard to realize when you're in danger. Especially if you're standing right in front of a trigger or binge-eating temptation, and you start to feel the urge building up. This doesn't mean that you should spend the whole day thinking about binge-eating urges. This would be devastating for your progress against the disease because if it's all you think about, you've already lost half the battle. You must find the awareness balance. If you start feeling anxiety, if you feel the slightest sign of a binge-eating urge building up, you should be able to identify it and start your defense mechanisms right away.

The idea to stop a binge-eating episode once you feel your urge seemed like something impossible. Once you've let that urge inside of you, you've lost the battle. Sooner or later, you're going to have to binge. You might as well start planning how you'll do it. Life doesn't have to be that way. We're not slaves of our disease. It can be hard, but it's not impossible to stop a binge-eating episode. You just have to change your mindset and delay the start of the binge.

So you already know that you have the urge to binge-eat. There's a chance that it will go away if you find a way to delay it. So if you're home watching the TV and you start with the binge-eating urge, you might benefit from keeping yourself occupied, especially if it's away from the kitchen and any possible source of food. Do some yoga, meditate, or take a walk through the forest. Forcing yourself to do something other than eat is possible before you start the binge-eating episode, and if you keep at it, you'll feel the urge slowly fading away.

You can also try to replace your thoughts with something else. If you're almost done, the disease is asking you to binge, and you've already lost hope. It may help if you try to change the topic of conversation in your mind. If you're thinking about the food that you're going to get in just a couple of minutes, you should try thinking about the reasons why you can't do that. Perhaps you can't afford those cheeseburgers (even if you can). Maybe you're too busy right now to start binge-eating (even if you have the spare time). Perhaps thinking about everything that you've done so far, the way this disease affects your family, your health, and how great you've been avoiding the binge-eating episodes up to this moment might be able to save you. Don't give up; fight the urge until the last moment. Fight smart, know your disease, know yourself, and know that not everything is lost once you feel the urge to binge-eat.

If after all of this you fall in a binge-eating episode, that's alright. First of all, try not to feel bad about yourself. After all, if stopping those binge-eating episodes was so easy, Binge-Eating Disorder wouldn't be the most common Eating Disorder there is. I know that this may feel impossible, but even at this point, there is something you can do to stop the binge-eating episode. You must take control of your binge-eating while it's happening. All you need to do is to eat willingly. You know that feeling of having an out-of-body experience during your binge-eating episodes. You're in autopilot. It's all happening in a sequence that's not controlled by you. You're too busy trying to make it stop, but your body won't do it. There's no use; you're already a disappointment. You're not worth the effort to end it. It's almost impossible to take control of your binge-eating episode this way. It's a lot easier to do it by eating willingly. I know it may sound like the opposite of what you should do, but if you willingly take your binge-eating episode in the same direction it's going, you will eventually turn off the autopilot, and it's you at the wheels.

So you're on your binge-eating episode. You're stuffing bite after bite of snacks, and you're doing it willingly, but you're still doing it. Obviously, that's not what you're looking for. Now you have to identify the exact moment when your binge-eating urge is going down so you can stop it. There's a moment during your binge-eating episode in which you've had enough food to feel good. You're probably not hungry anymore, and the food doesn't taste as great because you've already satisfied the craving. Finding this moment is hard. It takes some time and practice, but once you learn how to do it, you can stop your binge-eating episodes with a simple "alright, I've had enough of this, I think I'm good." That's it, that's all it takes. I know it's a halfway victory because you still ate. You still fell in the binge-eating episode. I understand that, but eating half a bag of

Doritos is better than eating the whole bag, going over to ice cream and opening another bag of Doritos to keep on the cycle. After you've done this enough, you'll start to gain confidence, and confidence is priceless when you're a binge-eater. Knowing that you're no longer a helpless victim of the disease, that you're able to fight back, is great for your self-esteem, and it helps with your previous conception of yourself as someone with no self-control whatsoever.

It should be noted that it is easier to stop a binge-eating episode in the early stages, and the best way to stop them overall is prevention. If you follow the rest of the recommendations in this book, you'll achieve a healthier way of life that will ultimately stop the urges from being born. And once you're in danger, it's easier to stop a binge-eating episode at that point than to do it during the binge. What I mean with this is that you shouldn't trust yourself so much that you'd think it doesn't matter you're in a danger zone, or if you're surrounded by my triggers, because you feel like you can stop any binge-eating episode just before it happens. The better moment to stop a binge-eating episode is before you have the urge. If you're in danger, or if you're starting to feel the urge, you should jump on the developing binge right away.

Working on your mental health is the best way to heal from this disease. If your mind is at ease, if you're not developing any new anxieties, your defenses against this disease are bulletproof.

Chapter Eleven

Group Therapy

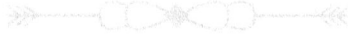

There's comfort in knowing that you're not alone. Right now, information about Binge-Eating Disorder was everywhere. It is a lot easier to do some research about this disease and to find people that are suffering from it. It is known that this disease is more common than Bulimia Nervosa and Anorexia Nervosa. Binge-Eating Disorder is a big deal, and we're all paying attention to it.

Back then, this was not the case. As a binge-eater, sometimes, I felt as if I had a new disease with no possible treatment. It was stepping into the unknown. Everyone knew about Bulimia Nervosa and Anorexia Nervosa, but no one knew about Binge-Eating Disorder. I had no way to foresee what was going to happen to me and no one to compare to.

This situation ended in my first group therapy session. I was very happy to find out that there were others out there who were the same as me. They all suffered from Binge-Eating Disorder, and some of them were already better. There was a way out of this dark pit. They were already walking that path. It was possible to survive this disease. It would not be the end of me.

I could see myself in the story of William. William was a fellow binge-eater. He was two years younger than me, and he used to sneak out of football practice to eat a bag full of candy bars in the lockers room. His teammates found out and made fun of him, which only made things worse. He felt as if his body was moving on his own whenever he binged, and I'm sure that I can relate to that. It is a terrifying experience. His binge-eating episodes got so bad, his life was so unbalanced, the bullying was so terrible, and the shame was so unbearable that he swallowed a whole bottle of pills trying to end it.

His story shook me to my bones because I know that I was close to going there. I was close to ending my life before I decided to turn things around. It might have been me just as well as it might have been him. Luckily, nothing happened to him. His family found him and took him to the hospital, so he was saved. After that experience, he decided, along with his family, to get professional treatment. He's much better now, on his way to recovery. He's grateful to be alive, and we're all glad we got to meet him.

I met Caroline, and she made me realize how lucky I was to have Alex. Caroline was a 29 years old woman recently separated from a man named Peter. Peter had a drinking problem. They were in love since high school, and she suffered from Binge-Eating Disorder, to which he didn't help much. He used to get drunk and say nasty things to her. He would disappear from their house for three days straight without saying a word to her. She just stayed there during these days, utterly consumed by anxiety. Whenever they had to get together with their friends and family, she was scared that he would get drunk and make a scene. The anxiety hours before that absorbed her, getting to the point where she had trouble breathing. Of course, all of this anxiety pushed her towards binge-eating episodes. She had a rough time, felt embarrassed, and then she would binge more.

This happened for four awful years until she finally left that man. Only then was she able to start getting treatment. She had to leave that house, go back to live with her parents, and be straight and open with them. She was a hard binge-eater. She didn't want to do it anymore. She needed help. Her marriage was a failure, which is why she never allowed herself to bring a baby to that home. Her parents helped her, just like my parents helped me, and she was able to recover. She's better now. She's not binge-eating as much, and she's not as consumed by anxiety as she used to be.

Robert taught us a lot about the importance of being healthy. He is a fellow binge-eater that's suffering from Type 2 Diabetes Mellitus. He's not the only one with Diabetes Mellitus in his family, so he'd always known that he was at risk of developing that disease. As if Binge-Eating Disorder wasn't bad enough. He got the diagnosis of Type 2 Diabetes Mellitus when he was 29 years old. Back then, he was obese, and he had to change the way he lived if he wanted to survive. Of course, it took a lot of work, and he is at a disadvantage because of Binge-Eating Disorder. It took him a lot of hard work and discipline, but he's alive thanks to it. He lost part of his right foot, which was a huge blow for him, but he's able to walk thanks to a prosthesis and special footwear. Thankfully he has the support of his family. He's living one day at a time. He is extremely careful, and he takes his treatment very seriously, both his medical treatment for Type 2 Diabetes Mellitus as well as the psychological treatment for The Binge Eating Disorder. He's doing alright. He's keeping his blood glucose levels normal, so if he keeps this up, he should be able to live a long and happy life.

Mary and Barbara taught me the dangers of binge-eating as a family. They both came from a huge family of people suffering from overweight. They were both obese. They'd been extremely overweight their whole lives, and it all started at home. Eating this much is normal in their family. Their parents are both that way. They spend about two hours eating dinner, and then they go and turn on the TV with a platter full of snacks in front of them. They're not sure if everyone in their family is suffering from Binge-Eating Disorder, but almost everyone suffers from obesity. Their parents, uncles, and cousins do; it's a part of their family traditions. They're all accustomed to eating huge amounts of food and to being overweight. They don't care about it very much. Mary and Barbara were with us because they wanted to change. They wish to be able to bring their mother and father to the therapy someday, but right now, they don't want to recognize there's something wrong with the way they live.

In order to start recovering from Binge-Eating Disorder, Mary and Barbara had to move out of that house filled with triggers and temptations. Some days, they ate a family size pizza with a 2L bottle of coke and a slice of apple pie each. Some of you may call this a strong binge-eating episode, but over there at their house, they just call it dinner. Binge-Eating Disorder can be more dangerous and aggressive if it's supported by your whole environment. Start thinking about yourself for a moment. What do you think that would've happened with your Binge-Eating Disorder if it was shared by your whole family?

Joe was a shining beacon of hope for everyone at the group therapy. He was a 45 years old man. He wasn't even fat. He'd recovered almost completely from Binge-Eating Disorder, and he was coming to these sessions mostly to help us get to where he is right now. He's very kind. He looks healthy, and he'd managed to stay free of binge-eating episodes for eight months now. Last year, he only had three of those.

Joe showed us that there is hope. Binge-Eating Disorder is not a death sentence. He went through the same things we're suffering right now, and he came out victorious. He's part of the reason why I decided to write this book, knowing him really helped me have hope, and you need to believe that you have a chance at victory if you're going to give it your all against this illness. I expect to be able to transmit this confidence and hope to you. Just as Joe is better, I am better. I'm telling you how I got better, and I know that you could be better too.

No matter who you are, group therapy is a positive experience. You should try it too; no one should be alone in this fight.

Chapter Twelve

Diabetes and Binge Eating

Some studies point out that approximately 12% of the people suffering from Binge-Eating Disorder are also suffering from Type 2 Diabetes Mellitus. I've seen this through my friend Robert on group therapy, and it's a very dangerous situation. Diabetes Mellitus is a disease that must be taken seriously. Sadly, there's no cure; people with that condition spend the rest of their lives on medication, food restrictions, and going to a doctor periodically to check on themselves. Type 2 Diabetes Mellitus is perfectly capable of taking your life if you're not careful, so this is something you shouldn't take lightly.

First of all, my advice to you is to investigate your family. Your risk of getting Type 2 Diabetes Mellitus is higher if a member of your family has it. So if a parent, sibling, uncle, grandfather, cousin, anyone from your family has it, and you're overweight, you should check your blood glucose levels with your doctor constantly to rule out the possibility of developing the disease. This is especially the case if you're obese and eating poorly (way too much sugar).

If you find yourself drinking more water than you used to, that's a symptom of Diabetes Mellitus. Another symptom is to urinate constantly. If you start going to the bathroom constantly, you should be worried. The other two main symptoms are weight loss and an increase of appetite, which are harder to detect when you're suffering from Binge-Eating Disorder. Being constantly hungry, eating more than you used to, more than a normal person, is already a part of your life and could easily be attributed to the eating disorder. And if you're doing things right, if you're recovering from the disease, you should also be losing weight. This makes it hard to think of Type 2 Diabetes Mellitus just from weight loss. Nonetheless, if you're losing weight and you know that you're still doing things wrong, perhaps you should put a pin on that and go to your doctor to check how you're doing.

Definitively, being diagnosed with Type 2 Diabetes Mellitus is bad news no matter who you are, but they're terrible if you're also a binge-eater. As if life wasn't hard enough just because of that. Avoiding sugar is extremely hard for us, considering that we usually lack discipline and self-control. That's something we all have to keep in mind because it is possible to avoid developing Type 2 Diabetes Mellitus. We just have to take care of yourself. I know that's not easy for us, but we're talking about our health, our lives could be at risk, so we shouldn't take the threat of Type 2 Diabetes Mellitus lightly.

Early medical detection is possible; you can even spot the disease before it is fully developed. If you start developing insulin resistance, you're in the early stages of Type 2 Diabetes Mellitus. You must make some major changes in your life, and you may need some medication, but if you start treating it at this point, your life expectancy is a lot higher. On the other hand, if you spot the disease when it's fully developed and you're unable to produce insulin, things don't look good to you.

If you've developed the disease, if you go to the doctor and receive the diagnosis of Type 2 Diabetes Mellitus, there's a couple of things that you should do as a binge-eater. First of all, both your doctor and your therapist should know about this situation. The doctor that diagnosed you with Type 2 Diabetes Mellitus should know that you suffer from The Binge Eating Disorder, and your psychiatrist, psychologist or therapist should know about the Type 2 Diabetes Mellitus. Also, your family should know too. Robert had the support of his family. They helped him avoid binges by avoiding food with high levels of sugar. Perhaps not everyone has a family willing able to provide such great help, but you should at least try. Nobody wants to lose their loved one, especially to such an awful disease. It is unlikely that you won't get any kind of help.

Type 2 Diabetes Mellitus doesn't mean that you will start eating less. If you're following my recommendations (and, most likely, the orders from your therapist), you should be eating five times per day. You shouldn't stop doing this. After all, it's the only way to avoid binge-eating episodes. As long as your blood glucose levels are normal, there's no need for you to stop eating. Besides, you should avoid low glucose levels, so starving is not advisable at all.

If you want to snack, there's a lot of available choices for you. Always speak to your doctor about what you should or shouldn't eat, but you'll likely be surprised by how little you have to change your diet. What should you do if you have a special love for ice cream? Well, there's ice cream for diabetic patients, it has no sugar. I've never tasted it, but Robert said it was alright. He had some a couple of times each week, and he was able to keep his glucose levels straight.

Do you remember what we talked about in the eighth chapter? As binge-eaters, we tend to have black and white thinking. If you start separating your food by good food and bad food, you'll probably end up feeling terrible if you have a taste of the bad food. A bad mood is a trigger for a binge-eating episode. In order to avoid this, you should keep track of your blood glucose levels. Maybe a peanut butter and jelly sandwich isn't as deadly as it seems if you check your blood glucose levels afterward, and they're normal. Checking your glucose levels will keep your eyes on the real danger, and you won't feel guilty after a minor slip if you find that it did no harm. This way, you can be sure of which kind of food you can eat without further advancing the disease.

Having Type 2 Diabetes Mellitus and Binge-Eating Disorder may sound like a very hard situation, but it's not a death sentence. Work hard, make an effort, and have faith; everything is going to be alright.

Chapter Thirteen

Helping as a Friend

Maybe you didn't get this book because you are suffering from Binge-Eating Disorder. Perhaps it's someone close to you that's sick, and you want to understand them, to be able to help. If that is the case, this chapter is for you.

Friends and family can be really helpful. You can make a difference in the life of your loved one. I know that I received help from my parents and my family. I'm very lucky to have them with me.

If you're reading this book, that means you're one step ahead from most people who want to help someone with a Binge-Eating Disorder. You know a lot more than the average citizen. You know what works and what doesn't, so you should be aware of what to advise them (especially if they haven't read this or any other book about their disease).

If you know that your friend has this disease, then he or she probably has already told you about it. Your friend has made an effort to reach out to you, so they're already looking for help from their loved ones. If he or she had talked to you about this, asking for your help, but you're the only one, and you know that the family is not aware of Binge-Eating Disorder, you should encourage your friend to tell them. No matter what kind of family it is, they should be aware of it. Keeping things secret is a way to add stress and anxiety to an already precarious situation.

Don't even try to get them on a diet. If you see them having such an idea in their heads, you should talk them out of it. Diets can be catastrophic for someone suffering from Binge-Eating Disorder, as we've already discussed. So if you want what's best for them, you'll look at them in the eyes and tell them that a strict diet is not the way to go. Instead, you know that a full diet, a planned diet is much better. They shouldn't waste time running after diets from fashion magazines that are intended for models. They should aim to eat like a normal person. We must go for five meals per day, aiming for rather healthy choices without starving.

You should be careful about how you speak and the things you speak about. Your friend doesn't need to have a conversation about their body, bodyweight, figure, clothing, diet, anything. Body shaming can be fatal for someone suffering from Binge-Eating Disorder. Trust me; we know we don't look great. Quite frankly, the chances are that we don't like how we look, but having someone to remind us that is the opposite of help. It's sinking us in our own misery.

Shield them from the negativity as much as you can. Inviting them to come over to watch America's Next Top Model should already strike you as a bad idea. Going out together with friends that you know are likely to make negative comments is even worse. It may sound overly dramatic to think this way, but it's the truth. If you want to help your friend who's struggling with Binge-Eating Disorder, you should put an effort and shield him or her from the negativity.

You may feel compelled to motivate your friend, but sometimes it's more harmful than beneficial. If you do it through threats such as "if you binge-eat again, we won't go to the movie theater for this whole year," or "you'll have to look for another one for support because I'm done helping you if you do it one more single time." Any kind of threat is negative. It won't help your friend at all. It will rather put pressure on them, and not in a way you would want them to. As we've already gone through this earlier in this book, the pressure will only make your friend think more about binge-eating. Having it present in their minds will increase the chances of another binge-eating episode. Besides, they will feel even worse after they binge because now they're letting you down. They are losing you somehow. Add that feeling to the shame of binge-eating, and you'll have a cocktail for a new episode.

I don't think there's anyone out there going through a mental illness that likes to be compared to others. I don't want to know about that friend of yours who struggled with cancer, recovered, lost his speech, and how he's capable of being happy in spite of that whilst I'm right here feeling miserable. I don't want you to tell me, "you know, you should feel lucky; there's a ton of people out there that wishes to be as fine as you are." Needless to say, it would be even worse to say something along the lines of "look at her, she also suffers from Binge-Eating Disorder, and she looks thinner and prettier than you."

This far ahead, I can't imagine that you would need me to tell you this, right?

If you want to help them, you should listen to them and try to understand how they feel. It's a lot easier to feel like you're not alone when there's someone who understands you. I know you can't read minds, and you're not going through the same hardships as we are, but you could still make an effort and try to get it. It goes a long way just to say, "I understand why you may feel this way." It's positive for us because it's validating. We at least know that we're not in the wrong for feeling this way, and that helps a lot.

The opposite of this would be to listen to how we feel and then trying to correct us, stating that we should feel another way instead. It is not helpful at all if I'm upset because I wanted to lose weight, and your answer is, "I think you should be happy because you didn't gain any weight." Something like "there's no reason for you to be this sad, you should be glad because..." is not helpful. If that's your idea of helping, I beg you to reconsider. This will only make us feel worse. Not only are we feeling the way we feel, but we're also wrong for feeling that way. Abnormal, inadequate, an outsider, shameful, an embarrassment, the perfect ingredients to a new binge-eating episode.

Earning specialized knowledge is an absolute plus if you want to help a friend or family member with Binge-Eating Disorder. Just the fact that you are reading this book proves that you're willing to go the extra mile. That's great, and I'm really happy for you and the person you care for. And yet, if you're willing to go this far, you should also consider getting professional counseling about the disease. Just as your friend needs professional help, he or she would benefit from you going to a professional therapist or counselor. This way, you can understand what he or she is going through. My husband did this a long time ago, and I could tell the difference.

Living with someone with a mental disease can be mentally and emotionally exhausting. I would know because I could tell whenever Alex was stressed, frustrated, or just plain tired. It made me feel terrible. Sometimes the best thing you can do is to take care of yourself. Alex's counselor advised him to take some time for himself, to recharge his batteries, so to speak. He spends a couple of hours each week playing videogames. Once per week or every two weeks, he likes to go out to a bar and drink beer with his two best friends (sometimes they come over to the house, and then he can do both, playing videogames whilst drinking beer). And if he doesn't have the time because he's buried in his work, listening to his favorite music can also be helpful. Just take care of yourself; you can't help anybody if you need to be taken care of.

Finally, no matter how great you think you are, you shouldn't try to take your friend's problems and pretend that you're able to solve them. This one is probably common to every mental illness out there. The idea that you can be somebody's savior is something that only happens in kid's stories. We're carrying a huge burden by ourselves. We're the ones that know it better than anyone else. Pretending that you can come, take that weight off our shoulders with your help, and turning our lives around all by yourself may be a little naive. The intention is good, but it is not possible. By the end of it, you may end up feeling resentment towards your friend because "in spite of everything you've done for him/her, it still isn't enough." That only happens because you've placed an unrealistic goal upon your friend. You've both failed to accomplish it. After this, after falling short, you're upset about failing. On the other hand, your friend probably feels the pressure. He or she may feel bad for failing, and when you add everything else, the results are the opposite of what you wanted.

Being there for your friend is not that hard. You just need to know how to do it. The best thing that you could do is to avoid harming your friend. If you manage to avoid hindering your friend, you're already doing more than most if you learn how you may be able to help your friend and do some good on his fight against Binge-Eating Disorder.

Your friend will love you for this. It is priceless to get the right kind of help.

Chapter Fourteen

Suicide Risk

If you want to know whether you are at risk of committing suicide, sadly, the chances are that concern comes from a bad place. If, on the other hand, you're reading this book to find out how to help a friend or family member suffering from Binge-Eating Disorder, God bless you. You're worthy of praise, and your friend is going to need every bit of help that he or she can get.

People with Binge-Eating Disorder, just as much as people with Bulimia Nervosa, are always at risk of committing suicide. We lack self-control, and we can be very impulsive. So whenever we're feeling awful, there is a chance that could lead to suicide.

Just think about the way an intrusive thought can really take us to do something we don't really want to. When we're already aware of the disease, and we want to stop the binge-eating episodes, that's not a lie. It's not a case of "you say you don't want to, but very deep, at the bottom, you really do." That's an oversimplification of what's going on inside our minds. Our biggest wish is to stop doing this to ourselves, to stop gaining weight. We don't want to keep feeling shame whenever we fall and binge-eat. We absolutely try to avoid it. It's just a moment of weakness because of the disease.

What do you think that happens when those thoughts start to suggest an alternative way out of that mess we're calling a life? Do you believe that we will be able to control ourselves forever? That's a very dangerous thought, and it is sad. It saddens me to think about those who were wise enough to get help but didn't receive any because no one believed they were at risk of killing themselves. When you suffer from Binge-Eating Disorder, you should always take this seriously, and if you're friends with someone suffering from that disease and you see one of these signs, you should take them to professional help immediately.

For example, if someone with a Binge-Eating Disorder speaks about wanting to disappear, that's a red flag. Conversations about wanting to leave for good, to sleep forever, about not having a reason to live, are all red flags and should be taken seriously. If they start talking about being a burden to the rest, to those they love, about not wanting to go on because of the disease, you should be worried.

People suffering from Binge-Eating Disorder may be impulsive, and as so, can be reckless. If they have that kind of personality, they will indulge in risky behaviors such as abusing alcohol, cigarettes, drugs, etc. But, if the person affected by the disease is not like that, and then they start behaving that way that is a red flag. If your friend starts drinking and smoking a lot, and they start with other reckless activities, with no disregard for their personal safety, you should have a deep talk with them.

Mood swings are also a cause to worry. Any mood impairments should be noticed as a possible red flag for suicide risk. If there's an increase in anxiety, anger, depression, and isolation, that's a good reason to be worried. Not every mood impairment should be interpreted as an increase of suicide risk, but it may be related to suicide risk if the mood swings are sudden, especially if you see the rest of the signs.

If those suffering from Binge-Eating Disorder start withdrawing from social activities, that's a red flag. If they start making up excuses to avoid going out with their friends, if they would clearly rather spend time alone in their rooms than go out, that's a reason to worry, especially if they weren't that way before. For example, I have always been an introvert. I never had many friends, and when I had Susan, sometimes I wanted to spend time alone in my room instead of hanging out with her. This is all about changes in behavior. If your friend used to be more outgoing and now he or she is passing on your dates, you should be worried.

If your friend starts to talk about death, to die, or to go as far as to say goodbye for no apparent reason, that is a major red flag. This one is pretty specific. You should always look for this kind of behavior. If you find it, please take it seriously. People with such clear signs should be monitored by their family. They should be aware of the risks, and they should look for professional help. The Internet is full of stories about people who talked about depression and suicide before doing it. People overcrowded by suicidal thoughts are looking for help. Talking with their friends and family about it is one of the most common behaviors you may find. By the end, those who tell these stories regret they didn't pay attention at the time. I'm sure you don't want to be like that too.

Finally, if by any chance you find out that your friend is sort of planning ways to commit suicide that is possibly the biggest red flag. If you check their browser's history and find that they're looking for ways to kill themselves, you should jump over that immediately. People get hospitalized for this kind of behavior. They're usually in such danger of committing suicide that they shouldn't be left alone without professional care.

You know your friend or familiar suffering from Binge-Eating Disorder. If you know of a previous attempt to commit suicide, you should always be on the lookout for another one and never let your guard down. Statistically, those who have already tried to commit suicide are more likely to try again. They need special help and care. Please, don't leave them alone.

I know that all of this may seem too much for some of you. It may be exhausting to care for someone that's so vulnerable. Not everyone is up for this task, and that's ok. I understand completely. I wouldn't blame you for it, but if you really care for that person in your life suffering from Binge-Eating Disorder, you should look after them. If you do, I believe that you've earned your place in heaven.

Chapter Fifteen

Will Love Save You

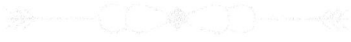

It's raining outside. The room is filled with 90's rock and pop music from the stereo, and our protagonist lays crying over her sofa; tormented by a disease that she never asked for, that's proving to be way more than she could handle. The table in front of her is filled with bags of chips and bowls with ice cream and cookies, and she's eating them, tears running down her cheeks over her snacks. There's a couple of knocks on the door. At first, she doesn't answer, but the person outside doesn't give up. The bangs at the door get a little bit harder, making sure to announce that person's presence outside. Our protagonist looks up with her makeup watered down from her tears, spreading as far as her cheekbones. She stands up and goes to meet the hero of the story. Sure enough, he's there; he brought roses and a bottle of wine. He's here to tell her that no matter what she's going through, they'll be going through it together. There's nothing that she can do to send him away. The scene ends with a kiss. Our hero holds the protagonist in his arms, and as she lets go, she lets the chips she was holding slip through her fingers, falling to the ground. The story of a charming prince's kiss that will make the curse go away is as old as time. It has been represented the same way with mental diseases, now, is this real? Is this what happens in the real world?

I can't talk about everyone's experience. I can only tell you how it was for me. I met Alex after I moved to a new high school. I was still very overweight, introvert, and I didn't trust any of my classmates after my last experience in the other school. I just wanted a fresh start where no one knew me, somewhere without bullying and nastiness. Alex was also somehow an introvert. He always had his nose deep into a book during recess, so he started to notice me when we were both reading alone on our respective benches.

The first time he talked to me, I was scared. I wanted him to go away, and I may have answered in a harsh way, but somehow he managed not to take it in a bad way. A couple of days later, he got the courage to ask me for a date. He wanted to go with me somewhere we could eat ice cream. As soon as he said that, my face got red as a tomato. I also got scared that I could somehow overeat (God forbid, maybe I would have gotten so nervous that I could've ended on a binge-eating episode). I said yes to going out, but I suggested that we could go to my favorite park instead. It was pretty nice, and we could walk around it. It was autumn, so the weather was lovely, and the trees were all painted orange, brown and yellow.

He said yes. That first date was awkward because none of us talked too much, and then I realized that not talking wasn't as catastrophic as I thought. On our following dates, we discovered that we could spend time together in silence without feeling awkward about it. We would spend time reading next to each other and watching movies. I would sit by him at his place as he plays videogames. All of this happened as we slowly got more affectionate, more used to each other, just closer.

The end of that story is obvious enough. We're married, happily married as I may add, and we have two beautiful daughters. He's a great husband, my life partner, and pretty much aware of my Binge-Eating Disorder. He does his best to help. He supported me at every decision I made regarding our daughters and how we would raise them. He follows my diet, so it's easier for me to keep it, and sometimes he even exercises with me. In reality, he's everything I could have asked for. He's my knight in shining armor, ready to help me beat this monster that we're calling Binge-Eating Disorder. Even though all of this is true, I can't say that he was a decisive factor in my recovery.

When I met Alex, I was already fighting against this disease. I was going to therapy, eating healthier, doing my positive reinforcement, keeping my journal, etc. I was already on the way of getting better, and he just showed up in my life. Looking back on it, perhaps he was more attracted to me because of it. It may have been possible to see how I was on the way to getting better. Maybe I wasn't as blue and grim as I usually was. But yet, I still struggled with this disease, and I had to do most of this alone. For the hardest part, it was just me against Binge-Eating Disorder. It was lurking at every corner, just waiting for me to slip so it could take over and make me binge. Nobody was able to face that for me, and that was fair. I had to learn self-control, and that was impossible if I received help.

I never did tell Alex anything in the beginning. When I decided to take him home to meet my family, I made sure that nobody would say anything inappropriate to him about the disease, and they all agreed. Whenever I was having a hard time, I made sure to stay away from him. I knew that I was likely to binge-eat, and I didn't want to escape from him in the middle of the park so that I could stuff a couple of cheeseburgers, fries, and a milkshake.

He did bring something positive to my life, and with that, I can say it was a little bit easier to fight the disease. He made me feel appreciated, cared for and admired in a way that no one ever had made me feel before. You know that your family loves you, but in a way, they're sort of supposed to. Because of this, a part of you won't let that caring raise your self-esteem the same way that an outsider's care and appreciation would. This was invaluable, and I loved him for that, still do.

On the other hand, not everything is roses and honey in relationships. Any relationship can go south really fast. We all have our issues, our little fights, and it was hard for me. After I got used to his presence in my life, those days in which I was having trouble with him were not as great for my binge-eating episodes. Anything that made me feel terrible, worthless, ashamed of myself, or just bad overall was negative for my binges. And if I did end up in a binge-eating episode, the shame that I felt inside me made me feel worse. Then I was in binge-eating season all over again. It was as terrible as any other thing that could have gone wrong in my life. For example, wanting to dress up nicely for him, looking at myself in the mirror and finding out that I didn't look the way I wanted to, was always a disaster for me. Managing to look a little bit better just to see him and spending the whole afternoon together without him noticing was also really bad for me.

I didn't tell him anything about my disease until I felt like I was getting the handle of it. I didn't want to scare him off. When I told him he just took a long pause, then he shot question after question to me until he understood what I was going through as much as he could. He started to help me lose weight, and he started to eat healthy with me. That was a huge help. Eating Chinese food on our dates, for example, was a rather healthy choice, a lot better than pizza and nachos. He took this the best way he could, and I'll be forever grateful for that. I love him with all my heart.

Overall, Alex is a great guy. He always has been. The fact that no relationship is perfect doesn't mean that he was bad for me or anything. As for the question I wrote as the name of this chapter, I would always advise you to not rely on anyone but yourself. It is always nice to have help. You should try to get help from those close to you, and your significant other can really get to help, but he may be as much as he may not be. I remember from the time I spent in group therapy, I learned from my friend Caroline that a bad partner could really mess you up and push you toward Binge-Eating Disorder. If you do have their help, that's great, but if you don't, you should still do this for yourself. No one is going to be as affected by this than you. No one is going to work for this more than you. And definitively, no one is going to do this for you. You must do this for yourself.

Chapter Sixteen

Raising Your Offspring

I was terrified to have one of my daughters become like me. The sole idea of it made my heart sink. I wasn't as far ahead as I am right now in regard to this disease when I got pregnant with my first child, and this is what occupied 70% of my mind. I didn't want them to follow my steps, to end up like me.

After spending some time with Barbara and Mary on group therapy, I learned that this situation was dangerously possible. Binge-Eating Disorder can be a part of a family's culture or traditions, just like obesity, alcoholism, and any other bad habit of the sort. If it's something that's normal in your family, it can be much more aggressive and unavoidable. I didn't want them to turn out like me, to go through the same suffering.

Thankfully, none of them did. I will place here every measure that I took in that regard so that you can repeat them with your children. I'm sure that those of you who have children feel the same way as I do. You want to save them from binge-eating. Don't worry; it's entirely possible.

First of all, and I do believe that this is the most important measure that you can take, make sure that you give them enough love and affection. Feeling alone and rejected is very hard, no matter who you are. It can get to be really brutal. Having your family as a backup can really save your life. I was lucky enough to have constant love from my mother with me, and I still developed the disease, so I guess that may not be just enough to save everyone. Considering this, my husband and I both try really hard to show our daughters that we love them. We find the time to spend time with them. We constantly compliment them. Plus, we always pay attention to what they have to say and express.

Loving your children is great, but you must also make sure that your love doesn't come only in the form of food. I love food, and my girls love it too, so it's really tempting just to give them something tasty every time I want to make them happy or celebrate an accomplishment. If you think about it, that's very deep into our culture. We tend to go celebrate a nice restaurant every time something great has happened in the family. If one of your kids has just gone into high school, what do you do? You take them to their favorite pizza or burger restaurant. Did they win any contest? Are they the new chess champion in the school? What a better way to celebrate than to go and get ice cream? It comes naturally to us, but that doesn't mean it's the best.

If my daughters get good grades, or if they have a ballet presentation, I try not to praise them through a nice dinner with cheeseburgers. Instead, I take them to a movie, for example. They can have popcorns and candy bars and everything they want, but the main event is not the food. The spotlight falls entirely over the film. I take them ice skating, for example. They absolutely love it. They can go at it for hours at a time. And once again, I'm not showing them my love through food. I've found a better way to show it, a healthier way. I've avoided the mental connection between my love and food. I still cook a nice meal for them every now and then, but that's not the only way we're going to bond.

Part of my issues with food was that it almost felt like the love of my mother. Her love came to me first this way. She always made great meals for us with those homemade flavors that we all yearn from our childhood. They just made me feel great, and as I grew older, it became the only thing that made me feel good. She almost seemed to read my thoughts every time I was blue; then, she would come with freshly baked cookies to cheer me up. It sometimes came with a hug and a kiss on the forehead, but mostly there was no need for that. The meals already made me feel appreciated and cared for. Food was love; that's how I knew it before it started to be my enemy.

I love my mom, and I know she meant well, but I do recognize that this was a mistake. I was not going to make the same mistakes with my daughters, so I had to find new ways to express cheer them up and express my love. My daughters like to play videogames, so I make sure to find the time to play Mario Kart with them. They love to dance, so I play the piano for them as they dance in the living room. They love skating, so I take them ice skating on special occasions. We go to movie theaters, watch Netflix as a family, and find ways to spend time together. I know that it may be hard to find the time to do all of this, but you surely don't need to. As long as you find a way to express your love to your offspring that doesn't rely entirely on food, you're going to be fine. More importantly, your children are going to be fine too.

This one may be hard, and a little unfair, but I know that it's a lot less likely to binge-eat if you don't have issues with your body, which is easier to prevent if you're not overweight. I didn't want my daughters to be overweight. I didn't want them to go through the same things that happened to me, so I made an effort regarding that when I was raising them.

Here is what I did. I already understood how to lead a healthy diet, so I did that with my daughters. I was responsible for it. We went to a nutritionist to develop a plan that would allow them to stay in shape and grow healthy. They ate five meals. The sizes were proportionate to their age and weight (we had a scale to measure everything), and I managed to slip through a couple of rather unhealthy meals without getting them out of shape. They still ate pizza, ice cream, and snacks, but the majority of their food was healthy, and it was still good. I'm a great cook, just like my mother, so everything I did was good and tasty, but that may not be always enough. Kids eat through their eyes; if the food doesn't look good, you have to find a way to make it seem more appealing. Kids don't like broccoli, but they don't mind having cream with broccoli, potatoes, carrots, and chicken. Peas are often left aside on the dish, but if you serve it mixed up with the rice, add bits of carrots and peppers, and then it ends up being a colorful, cheerful, and delicious meal. It's not impossible to make them eat good food, but you just have to find a way.

I also found something that they liked to do that meant exercise. For your children, it may be baseball, football, soccer, Martial Arts, whatever they like the best. For my daughters, it was dancing. They love ballet, and it's great exercise. Almost everyone likes something that means moving around. If your kid just wants to play paintball or airsoft (just like my husband), that also works. It doesn't matter what it is as long as they do it a couple of times each week. That will help them in so many ways through life. Being healthy is extremely advisable, and not being overweight is great for self-esteem.

You have to be careful not to go to the opposite end of the spectrum. Your kids should never feel like they're on a diet, much less be afraid of gaining weight. And if they are, they must never, no matter what, feel self-conscious about it. Don't ever tell your kids that you shouldn't eat something because that something makes you fat. You should never introduce that fear into their young minds, that thought may even provoke a different kind of eating disorder.

So you must have your children on a healthy diet, get them to any extracurricular activity that allows them to exercise regularly, and still allow them snacks because there's no way to have happy childhood without candy bars and treats. Try to get them to be healthy, to stay healthy, but don't make it hard on them. You can't be too strict about it, or you'll end up provoking another kind of eating disorder.

You should also be careful about their education experience. I was bullied pretty badly when I was young, all the way through high school. I know how hard that can get, how much it can hurt, and I know better than to let them go through the same awful situation I had to endure. You can't go to the school with them, neither should you fight their battles for them, but that doesn't mean there's no way to look over their shoulders. Before I got them to school, I made sure that their policy about bullying was strict. I also talked to their teachers regularly just to check on my daughters, asking the school staff to keep an eye on them. I can't say for sure if they suffered from any bullying, but to the best of my knowledge, they didn't. They also didn't develop an eating disorder.

I also made sure that they knew how beautiful they really were. The perception of beauty is subjective, beauty is in the eye of the beholder, so if I taught them to believe that they were beautiful. They would really feel that way about themselves, and there's no bigger win than that. All you have to do is to tell them that they're pretty. It is not that hard, simple and short comments such as "you look so cute in that dress" and "I just love your hair today" will do the trick. Of course, you shouldn't ever teach them that they're beautiful by demeaning the rest. I wanted my daughters to be confident without being the same as those who gave me a hard time in school. We taught them to respect everyone else around them. For as much as they feel pretty, it doesn't mean that they feel prettier, better, or superior to everyone else.

My daughters are a little older by now, and they turned out fine. They do ballet, go to school, and by all appearances, live a happy childhood. They have a healthy weight, don't binge, and as far as I'm aware, they're not victims from bullying at school.

It can be done. It is possible. As someone who suffered from Binge-Eating Disorder, I'm telling you that you could have your kids, raise them, and still save them from being like you.

It's way too good to see my daughters shining with the light of their happiness and health. I'm so proud of them.

Chapter Seventeen

Making Peace

We're finally here. I have already taught you almost everything you should know to survive this. Every tip that I've gathered that helped me through the beginning of this disease, and those that I'm sure I would've loved to have when I needed them.

You're almost set. You can go now and heal your relationship with food. There is no need to see it as your enemy as a part of your disease. A part of the healing process is to be positive, which is impossible if you're seeing enemies everywhere. You can't have something that you absolutely need to survive as your worst enemy.

My advice to you is to start eating as if it were a religious ritual. Your body is your temple. It is sacred, and you need to treat your food as the holy fuel that is going to keep you alive. This serves two purposes: First, after hating yourself so much, appreciating yourself and your body is a nice change of scenery; last but not least, it forces you to stay focused on the process of eating and to eat slower.

I believe that the most important effect, the one that creates a bigger change in your relationship with food, is to eat slower. I feel that every time that I'm on a binge-eating episode, my mind goes blank, then I start eating like a machine. I become like a wild animal without even noticing. During this sort of trance, I'm very aware of the food that I was eating; it just sorts of disappears before me. Forcing myself to eat slower makes me think of my food. I actually feel like I'm eating; every bite starts to matter.

When you eat slowly, you need less food to feel full. The more you chew, the more your brain believes that you're eating, the more satisfied you are. Focusing on every bite, taking less than a complete mouthful every time, and avoiding swallowing everything right after it hits your tongue all help in making you feel satisfied. Besides, when I take too much time eating, I feel less at risk of falling into a binge. One of its most important characteristics is that it happens during a short span of time. Eating at a slow pace has helped me to eat less, and to appreciate food for its quality rather than its size.

I know I said that was the most important effect you'll get out of making your meals a spiritual experience, but that doesn't mean that the other advantages should be left out. Ever since I was little, I never treated my body with respect. I wasn't proud of it. In reality, I was rather ashamed. I saw it with disgust, and all I felt for it was hatred. It always seemed to me like a curse. I just didn't deserve being this way, and no one should ever feel like this, especially a little girl.

When I started to work on my self-esteem, I used to do a lot of positive reinforcement, as you may recall from earlier in this book. It was good for me, but still, I didn't buy it 100%, especially at first. When I looked at myself in the mirror, I thought, "I am beautiful," and a very strong voice deep from within me said, "No, you're not."

You know how we are. We have a tendency to think in black and white, so I thought I was absolutely hideous. It felt horrible. Still, I tried to ignore that voice. Answering the disease is not the best way to defeat it. It's often stronger after that.

There is another way to answer this. Yes, you should say that you are beautiful, but you should also that no matter what, you look like you deserve affection. You deserve to take care of yourself and your body. Your body is your temple. When you start treating it that way, it gets easier to live with. And it is easier to believe, when you say that your body is your temple, the deep voice from within can only answer "no, it is not, it is hideous", and you can say "no matter what it looks like, it's still my temple, and it's sacred". The voice will have nothing to respond to this. Treating your body like your temple is easier if every time you eat, you treat your food as a gift for your body. It's ambrosia for the goddess that lives in my body; gold and pearls for the castle she lives in.

Treating your food this way will give it a new meaning. You will no longer be able to hate it. The food becomes your ally, something you need in order to charge your batteries and a proper offering for your temple.

Food needs to become something you're not terribly ashamed of. People shouldn't be tormented by their diets. Once you reach here, I want you to be able to forgive yourself if you eat something that's a little bit off your diet. So you had a slice of cheesecake with a ball of ice cream in one of your children's birthday party, and you're eating it with the rest of the mothers whilst the children are playing happily in the backyard. If the children ate the same thing, the chances are that they're happy because of it; you, on the other hand, are surrounded by women feeling guilty for eating this. It's ideal to avoid eating these rather unhealthy dishes, but that doesn't mean that you're not going to eat them again at never in your life. You'll most likely eat them, and if you do, you must do it with ease, at peace. After all, a single bite won't harm. Binge-Eating Disorder is so powerful because it rides over your shame and self-embarrassment. This needs to stop or else you'll spend the rest of your life at its mercy, always vulnerable to it, just a minor slip away from a new binge-eating episode.

Once you've got your life in order and you see results in your monthly measure of the scale, it's easier to make peace with the little snacks. You just have to focus on how much you deserve this, and after going through this, you do.

You'll reach peace when you're able to eat without feeling guilt or shame. Peace with food means being in peace with yourself. It loves yourself the way you are.

Conclusion

Thank you very much for reading up to this point. If you bought this book and you took the time to read it, there's no way that you're not going to get through this. You're already ahead of most people suffering from this disorder. You know that you are sick, you know what you have, and you know the right way to fight this and win.

What's left for you is to start applying this. I would advise you to start with your family and friends. Doing this on your own, even if you know exactly what to do, might be really hard. I know that you can get tons of help from them, and if you really feel like you won't, you'll most likely be surprised. There is somebody out there for everyone, even for the loneliest of us. I would even advise you to have them read this book. Those that are especially interested in helping you should know how to do it. They will understand you a lot better once they read this book.

After getting help from your family, your closest friends, and your significant other if you have one, you should get professional help. A psychiatrist would be my first choice, but maybe that's a bit expensive for everyone. Besides, maybe you feel like a psychiatrist is too much stigmatized, and you don't want to be perceived as "that lunatic that goes to a shrink." Well, first of all, I don't agree with that mindset. The stigma over mental illnesses is extremely unfair and uncalled for. Besides, nowadays, people perceive mental illnesses as normal. Still, if a psychiatrist is not the way you'd go, you can go to a therapist or a clinical psychologist. The only thing that matters is to do it.

You should also ask for group therapy. There is a way to get some of the advantages I described without actually going to group therapy. You could go to a forum and meet people with Binge-Eating Disorder, share stories, and gets that feeling that you are not alone. You could also go to binge-eating meetings or organize them in your city if you don't have any. Talking, being able to bond with another person that's going through the same issues you're facing is invaluable, but that's not the only thing you'll be getting at group therapy. During group therapy, you'll have a guide. Someone, there will be treating all of the members in the circle. You'll learn from watching another human being facing the same issues that you're facing, and you'll be forever grateful for them, for they will be your greatest teachers. In summary, get the professional help that takes you to group therapy.

These are the first two steps that you should take. They are the most meaningful, and they have the strongest chance to change your life. Nonetheless, that doesn't mean that it's the only thing you should do. At any given moment, but rather sooner than later, you should start with the little changes in your life. Start with the journal, the positive reinforcements, to befriend your illness, to keep a realistic diet, etc. All of these things really add up in the long run. This is what will ultimately save you.

I'm very excited about you! I'm so happy that you are going to take care of yourself and beat this thing! My heart is full of joy just by thinking on every single girl and woman out there just like me that passed through this and right now is ready to get better.

After writing this book for you, with your image in my head, I feel like I know you. I care for you and wish you the best.

Now you're on the path out of this maze, come meet me on the other side.

Resources

HYPERLINK "www.waldeneatingdisorders.com"

HYPERLINK "www.webmd.com"

HYPERLINK "www.healthline.com"

HYPERLINK "www.eatingdisorderhope.com"

HYPERLINK "www.eatingrecoverycenter.com"

HYPERLINK "www.psychcentral.com"

HYPERLINK "www.nationaleatingdisorders.com"

www.ingramcontent.com/pod-product-compliance
Lightning Source LLC
Chambersburg PA
CBHW050744030426
42336CB00012B/1651